TRIUMPH OVER HEPATITIS C

Lloyd Wright

PART 1:

HOW AMERICAN DOCTORS DEAL WITH HEPATITIS C.

THE PERSPECTIVE OF ONE PATIENT DETERMINED TO LIVE HEPATITIS C FREE.

PART 2:

THE REMEDY:

THE ALTERNATIVE MEDICINE SOLUTION THAT SAVED MY LIFE.

DISCLAIMER

The Reader or Purchaser of this book hereby acknowledges receiving notification in this Disclaimer that any opinions expressed herein are solely those of the company TRIUMPH OVER HEPATITIS C. None of the opinions expressed herein are to be relied on as statements of fact. Anyone having any questions regarding the success of the products described herein can contact TRIUMPH OVER HEPATITIS C at the phone numbers or email address noted below. Anyone who purchases either this book, or any of the vitamin supplements described herein, in reliance on either the book or the web site of TRIUMPH OVER HEPATITIS C, acknowledges that they are relying on their own investigation and not on any statements of opinion as to the success ratio of utilizing the treatments set forth in either the book or on the web site. The buyer of this book and/or purchaser of goods described herein acknowledges that they are making their own independent decision after discussing this matter with their current physician. No one should attempt to utilize any method of treatment set forth on either the web site of TRIUMPH OVER HEPATITIS C or in this book without first consulting their own personal physician for approval in utilizing the alternative health care methods discussed herein.

Publisher's Cataloging in Publication

Lloyd Wright.
  Triumph Over Hepatitis C / Lloyd Wright—3rd ed. 2nd printing
  pp. 303.
  Includes references.
  ISBN: 0-9676404-4-X

Illustrations by Annie Waterhouse
Typeset and Design by THE COPY STORE
Cover Design by Peri Poloni: www.knockoutbooks.com

Printed in the United States of America   2 3 4 5 6 7 8 9 10

TRIUMPH OVER HEPATITIS C
AN ALTERNATIVE MEDICINE SOLUTION
PUBLISHED BY
LLOYD WRIGHT
P.O. Box 6347
Malibu, CA 90264
Phone (866) Hep C Free - (866) 437-2373
Email - Lloyd@hepatitiscfree.com
Website - www.hepatitiscfree.com

This book is dedicated to Pattie,

for reasons that need not be explained here,

the men and women of Fire Station 56,

and to Bob Dylan for *Political World*.

CONTENTS

PART II – THE REMEDY

ACKNOWLEDGEMENTS

While it has been almost eight years since I began documenting the ballistic treachery that has plagued my life since my diagnosis of hepatitis C and my recovery, I continue to strive to shape a piece of written material that can help other people faced with this seemly impossible mission and to let them know that hepatitis C can be overcome! I stand alone in a world of non-believing medical doctors.

My special thanks go out to Irwin Zucker for bringing my quest to millions of Americans through radio and T.V. programs and encouraging me to attend the UCLA Festival of Books, New York and Chicago Book Conventions, and many additional educational programs.

A huge thanks to my staff, who answer phone calls from all those who call and deal with the huge amount of paperwork involved in what has become a 24-hour a day endeavor fighting "The Dragon."

Thanks to the special people who have practiced my Remedy and have called, e-mailed and written expressing gratitude and endless thanks for their normal liver panels and return to normal life!

My thanks to my readers, who can overlook the fact that I am not a doctor or a literary genius, just a person who found an answer.

Special thanks to Dr. Yeast de Villars, Dr. Miller, Dr. Nichols, Dr. John Finnegan, Dr. Ed Wagner and Dr. Debar Banker.

Finally, I would like to thank Dr. Roy for telling me to THINK. He wrote this word on a piece of paper and circled it. That paper is still on my refrigerator today. Dr. Roy's suggestions have transformed my life.

Lloyd Wright
June 2002
Malibu, California

INTRODUCTION

John Finnegan, N.D.

The health of the world population is deteriorating at an accelerating rate due to humankind's pervasive pollution of their environment, a depletion of nutrients in the soils and food, and an imbalance in our way of living. Yet in the midst of this darkness of our own creation there is the dawning light of special knowledge of herbs and nutrients. These herbs and nutrients give protection and healing to those who strive to live consciously and who are open to appreciating God's creations in nature.

Mr. Lloyd Wright has written an account of his journey from infection with hepatitis C to becoming hepatitis C free. He is a person who went to the extreme to conquer his life-threatening ailment. He diligently practiced all of the pertinent knowledge he obtained. Regardless of the peril necessary to acquire funds, Mr. Wright reached beyond the medical establishment of the 20th century to obtain the knowledge necessary to continue living.

The FDA's only approved drug for hepatitis C is interferon. The use of this isolated, single action drug creates imbalances in the body's digestive and immune systems as well as interferes with brain function, triggering a domino effect of dysfunction and deterioration throughout the entire body. Keep in mind, there is nothing more powerful or holistically designed than our own body's systems for growth, health, defense, and healing.

While the drugs prescribed by medical professionals are becoming less effective and more harmful, it is evident that there is a tremendous need for health practitioners to look to holistic, alternative methods that are effective against disease while at the same time strengthening the immune system and supporting the body's overall health.

Many people, including medical practitioners, feel that herbs are good for minor things, but they don't have the capacity to help the body fight serious diseases. In fact, there are many herbal therapies that have profound effects on curing even the most serious disease. Mr. Wright provides a valuable service by identifying these therapies in his book.

People and doctors rely on pharmaceutical solutions because this is what they know. Yet it was reported by the American Medical Association in 1998 that even when taken properly, prescription medicines account for 100,000 deaths each year and a million hospitalizations. We accept these pharmaceuticals as our "health care" treatments even though they can cause serious imbalances and harmful side effects that impact our quality of health and life.

Conventional medicine certainly has its place in crisis intervention when the body is traumatically hurt or seriously failing. However, nutritional and herbal therapies should certainly be considered and tried before resorting to invasive, costly medicines and treatments.

A lack of awareness and education, in addition to misinformation put out by both the pharmaceutical and the natural products industries, as well as poorly processed natural products have kept most of us in the dark about the proper use and possibilities for effective herbal remedies.

Mr. Wright's long and costly journey through the dark halls of conventional medicine led him to discover and try these herbal and alternative remedies. If he had not done so, he would be dead today.

John Finnegan, N.D. is a Doctor of Naturopathic Medicine, researcher, and author of 10 books presenting his work in the holistic health sciences. His previous works, *The Facts about Fats* and *Recovery from Addiction* have received widespread professional recognition.

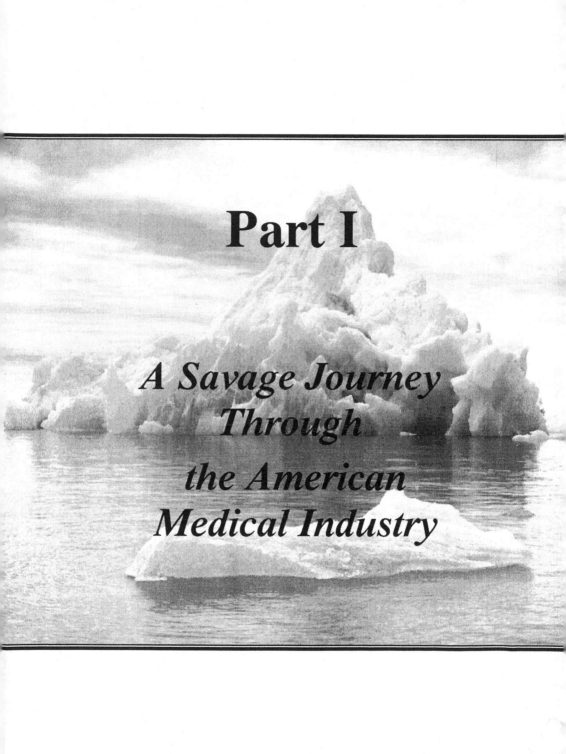

Part I

A Savage Journey
Through
the American
Medical Industry

THE GATES OF HELL

During the late summer of 1979, September 9th to be exact, I fell through the gates of Hell while operating my newly purchased John Deere tractor.

The "yellow monster" suffered catastrophic mechanical failure; the hydraulic reverse system had failed, summoning Lucifer himself. Backwards it thundered, flipped over, and launched me behind it as it went thrashing through the bushes and careened down a thousand-foot cliff.

I was crushed when the sixteen thousand pound defective John Deere tractor rolled over me on a very steep, remote site in the Santa Monica Mountains. There were no people or houses within miles. Blood gushed from my pants as if I were wading in it. My vision went black and white, or probably more like gray. I felt very peaceful, and lay down to die.

To my surprise, a lone horseback rider at a great distance had seen this happen. He had a small CB radio and made a call. Within several minutes a Medi-Vac helicopter landed. With much effort they carted me up the hill on a stretcher. All I remembered about what happened was that my guard dog, Jerome, leaped in the helicopter on top of my body and then began attacking my rescuers.

I woke up in Los Robles Hospital. I'm told it was the only hospital in the Western Hemisphere at that time with two hyperbolic chambers. This was experimental medicine to prevent crushed tissue from dying.

The surgeon on duty said my leg was broken in at least six different places, and my massive crush injury probably would result in kidney failure and death.

Over the next thirty days, I underwent nine major surgeries to reattach my leg. I received four blood transfusions and, unknown at the time, I also received a lethal dose of hepatitis C.

FIRST ENCOUNTERS WITH "HEALTH CARE PROFESSIONALS"

In 1983 my doctors took away my pain medication, Percodan. They said my liver was inflamed. I was in extreme pain and was told that I was going to have to learn to live with it. This news was a little hard for me to handle. I build houses and was in the process of creating a forty-acre avocado ranch. The doctors wouldn't give me any more drugs. Those doctors should be shot and wounded and left to flounder until death. Perhaps then they would understand why people who are in pain need painkillers.

They prescribed a mood elevator called Desyrel (Trazodone) HCI. In a few months, I was paranoid about

3

going to the local market, and I found myself in bed with a large woman and her daughter.

Seven years passed. My physician told me my liver count was a little high, but there was no cause for worry. Then in 1991, I was diagnosed with malignant testicular lymphoma – cancer. Oh joy, they were going to castrate me.

I frantically searched for and found a decent, honest doctor and he performed the procedure in an outpatient facility for twelve hundred dollars cash. Seconds before "putting me under," the doc handed me a form giving him the right to cut out whatever cancer he found. That meant I could wake up without "JR." Well, that's a wonderful way to "go under."

I was given morphine, my drug of choice, for signing away my "masculinity" for a plastic tube.

They prepared me for a shave. The lady who prepared me could have shaved a t-rex. She was very strong and capable, excellent with a razor; she was an absolute necessity when one's penis is at stake.

Twelve hours later I woke up on a bed in the middle of this sea of recovering patients; there was a row of beds in each direction for as far as I could see.

My first mission was to reach down and feel, hopefully, something that was there before. Thank God, "JR" was there. The right testicle didn't make it, but the left did.

The next crisis was that I had to urinate at least half a cup before they would let me out of this God-forsaken body part removal facility. Hours, I'd say six, and I just could not do it. Finally, I faked it with two drops of urine and half a glass of water. "JR" has functioned great ever since and, in fact, maybe better.

They gave me a few weeks to recover, a bottle of Percodan, and added instructions regarding no alcohol or sex for six weeks. My female sex partner was waiting for me when I got home. They must have used steel stitches, because that "she creature" did everything in her power to break them loose. I mean, imagine a bottle of Percodan, a case of Dom Perignon, and a wild, crazy Latino. "JR" went at it for days.

During radiation therapy, the oncologist told me my liver count was so high that I must be a serious alcoholic. I denied the charge. After therapy, he continued to monitor my liver count. At one point he said it was so high that I must be an intravenous drug user. I informed him that I had never stuck a needle in my body and my alcohol intake was negligible. After much debate, the oncologist tested me for hepatitis C. It was July 7, 1991.

The first type of hepatitis C test used was an inaccurate test, and it showed my result was negative. In September of that same year, however, the test for hepatitis C was perfected; but no one told me there was a new test or retested me!

Well now, here I was, my body crushed and nearly castrated. Then, as if that's not bad enough, my insurance company canceled my policy, and I didn't have any family to help me; they had all died from cancer, except my father. I truly love him, but he didn't make financial grants.

After two months of 180 rads of radiation a day, I couldn't function. I was supposed to eat well, but I didn't have any money. Ever pay cash to get neutered and radiated? Well, I got a real deal because I paid cash for the initial clipping.

The rads really took a toll on me though. I couldn't do anything except drive to and from the hospital, five days a week. It took one hour to get there, one hour to get back, and an eternity while I "got zapped."

5

During this time, I had much debate with my oncologist. First there was what he supposed to be my serious alcohol problem. I mean, he thought I was a "sterno user." He also suspected me of being an intravenous drug user, because my liver test scores were outrageous. I liked to party, but I didn't sit around drinking all day, and I never shot drugs.

This man, who was a radiation oncologist, had been a rocket scientist before becoming a doctor. Back in the 70's he worked on the space shuttle. One day he decided he wanted to "nuke" people instead. He spent some time in New Mexico, and bingo, he's an oncologist.

He knew nothing about blood transfusions or hepatitis. Apparently he didn't even know that the first hepatitis C tests performed were as accurate as Sitting Bull shooting an arrow at the moon.

The hepatitis C test wasn't perfected until September 1991, but did anyone ever think of retesting me? No! Did any doctor ever realize that my negative test result was the result of an unreliable test? Of all the doctors I saw, not one even knew anything about this until I saw a state-appointed psychiatrist/neurologist, who was working on the Gulf War Syndrome.

I saw this doctor four years after the first hepatitis C test when I was being reviewed for the second time for disability. The state thought I was crazy, because under the question regarding what sports I practiced daily, I finally wrote "masturbation." The first two times I had left this section of the form blank, as I was in no condition to practice sports, but then I decided this was an appropriate answer.

This brings me to my second encounter with the federal government. Broke and hungry, I figured I had paid Social Security all my life, more than most because I was self-employed. I've paid lots of property tax, and I went to the right welfare office for my zip code, right next to the Federal Building in Los Angeles.

I parked my car and walked to the door. Two large "uniformed officers" were on each side of a metal detector. I was frisked and felt up; I was the only white boy there and I think the "officers" really enjoyed this.

I got the forms, filled them out, and sat waiting for my name to be called.

A young black man sitting next to me began to laugh uncontrollably. After he slowed down, he sneaked a can of "Bud" out of his coat pocket and took a sip. So much for the metal detectors!

He said, "What's wrong with you white boy? You got shrimp for brains? You can't have an address and get nothing." Then he cracked up again. "White boy, you got shrimp for brains. You got to get another form. You can't have a bank account and get something from these fools. White boy, you got to get a new form. I'll help you. You got to lie. You got to lie or you get nothing. They don't give a rat's ass about your gonads. You got to tell them you got no home, no brains, no nothing and they got to believe you is crazy."

Well, I decided not to lie; and yes, he who lied got. I got nothing. So much for Social Security. I thought the federal government should shove off and fry in hell, at least as far as proclaiming that there was medical help available for anyone who needed it.

The federal government didn't help me in this crisis. I didn't make any money during this time, and I was suffering badly. The silent killer, hepatitis C, was working on me and no one knew it. The government sent me to a doctor in Los Angeles in late 1991 to be screened for Supplemental Security Income (SSI). He was a pulmonary

7

doctor, and I was sent there because of my liver and testicular cancer! I was very puzzled as to why they sent me to a "lung" doctor for my liver and testicular cancer.

He examined me and his advice was "stop taking vitamins A, C, D, E, and K, and your liver count will fall."

Was this why I paid taxes? Was this why SSI was developed?

This doctor had all my records. He knew about blood transfusions, and he knew about hepatitis C, didn't he? Then again, maybe he didn't.

I'm a contractor and I know my trade. When I paint the outside of a house, I don't use watercolors. My personal belief is that these fools who <u>practice</u> medicine should be paid less than I am, because <u>I'm not practicing</u>. I know my profession.

Don't get me wrong, I admire a good mechanic, which is all a good doctor can ever be. For the most part, fixing body parts is the only thing they learn how to do in medical school. They still can't cure viruses or the common cold.

I was dying from a yet unknown cause, and I was told to stop consuming vitamins! I was refused by Medi-Cal, and there were no other programs available for single white males between the ages of 21-65.

BLOOD BANK DIAGNOSIS

I felt like I had not recovered from radiation therapy for two years. I was subjected to 180 rads a day for two months over most of my lymph system, and I just never felt well again after that.

In 1993, I was building my own house. In the past, when I built a house (especially one of my own houses), I had loved it. I would work twelve hours a day and on weekends as well. Now I could not make it through the day. I was tired and sick. I complained, mostly to my primary physician, that I could no longer drink any alcohol at all because it made me sick, and he responded, "That's good. The stuff is bad for you anyway."

After three years of becoming more and more tired, breaking fingernails, my hair falling out, dizzy spells, and

9

having sweats at night to the point of my entire bed being soaked, the doctor told me I probably just needed a rest.

I went to a gastroenterologist, Dr. D. I ended up there because my dentist gave me an antibiotic that caused bleeding lesions in my colon. All my blood ended up in the toilet. He inserted a giant silver prod into my anal canal, devastating my posterior rectum for at least a year. He never even apologized. I was instantly considered a drug addict if I asked for any pain medication. I noticed several large books about the liver on his shelves, so I mentioned my high liver panel numbers from years earlier.

After extensive diagnoses, he decided that I had too much iron in my liver (see Iron Binding and Ferritin tests, pg 249), and I began having weekly phlebotomies. I went to a blood bank once a week and had my blood sucked out. It was supposed to be discarded as toxic waste.

Fortunately for me, one fine day someone screwed up and placed my blood with the donation blood and it was randomly tested. Two months later, the blood bank sent me a letter stating I could no longer donate blood because I had hepatitis C. What a surprise!

The first thing I did was to call the blood bank and ask for someone who could answer some questions. I was transferred to a technician, who said he knew quite a bit about hepatitis C. He graciously explained that I could expect to die from either hepatitis C or hepatocellular carcinoma, a complication of hepatitis C. He said there was no cure and I would suffer a slow death from internal bleeding and flu-like symptoms. It would be a long, slow demise, regardless of the path the disease took.

That was really exciting news!

Diagnoses given over the phone often inspire me. They lead me to believe that there are these small-minded fools presiding in offices all over the country just waiting to deliver some devastating news to the first person they can. It's like a collection agency that proclaims you're going to live under a bridge when they're through with you, for being a day late on your credit card payments.

I took my test results to two doctors, first, my general practitioner. I asked him what hepatitis C was, and what I should do about it? He said, "I don't know. Let me look into it, and I'll get back to you."

Then I went back to Dr. D. with my test results and asked him the same questions. I received the same answers, but he did get back to me right away.

He advised me that since I had no insurance, I should go directly to the county hospital. I assured him that was not an option. I was not about to let some county employee prolong my suffering or hasten my demise.

Then he told me about interferon alfa-2B recombinant, the only medication approved by the Federal Drug Administration (FDA) for hepatitis C at that time. He said it had some side effects, but nothing serious, and it had a cure rate of eighty percent. (Refer to Appendix A for information on interferon).

I was instructed to inject three million units of this medication in a different place in my body every other day. I went to the pharmacy and purchased a two-week supply: six vials for $692.00.

In just one week, I was transformed into a monster. My head was exploding. My brain was landing on anyone who was nearby. I'd cry; different parts of my body would sweat, and my head would be completely soaked, while my penis felt like it had icicles on it. I'd stay in bed for days. I couldn't function, and God help anyone who called on the phone. I reported my intolerance to the doctor; he cut my dose in half.

Meanwhile, in an attempt to conserve the outflow of my dwindling supply of cash, I applied to a program supported by the drug manufacturer and the government called Commitment To Care. This program was designed to help people without insurance who are in need of the (supposed) wonder drug, interferon. I received a really nice letter of rejection, indicating that anyone with a Malibu address did not qualify.

MEDICAL TORTURE AND INTERFERON NIGHTMARE

Dr. D. ordered a liver biopsy.

The doctor who performed the test told me that I wouldn't even know it had happened. Then he injected a needle about two feet long the diameter of an ink pen into my liver without any anesthesia. I swear that man will die and burn in hell. It was like being shot by a flaming arrow from a wild Indian. Later, I was told I wasn't given any pain medication because I was a cash patient.

As I lay there feeling like I was dying, the young and inexperienced doctor, who I'll call "Pocahontas," decided to give me a Percodan.

I want to know what these fools learn in school! Do they just stick needles in cadavers all day? This slime ball injected something the size of a primitive arrow into my side, guided it into my liver, and didn't give me any medication to dull the pain. Was one painkiller going to turn me into a heroin addict? Was the bastard afraid the Drug Enforcement Agency was going to jail him for intoxicating a patient? Perhaps it's just my karma that I'm supposed to suffer?

I can't understand for one minute what goes on in the heads of those mechanics, i.e. doctors, who think of themselves as little "gods."

Why did the government pay drug companies to develop the drugs? Was it so only the drug dealers could profit or so the insurance companies could rake in hundreds of dollars per pill?

I think these small-minded "gods" should be required to be patients themselves, and when they are in class, have their classmates stick "arrows" in their sides without medication. Let them beg for death. Actually, considering their mentality, they might end up being supporters of Dr. Kevorkian, rather than conscious of the need for drugs.

The most important thing to understand is that cash patients are treated differently than insurance and welfare patients. Welfare patients are probably given some generic non-narcotic drug such as Vicoden; unless it is a woman with a child, in that case she will probably get morphine and childcare.

The patients with insurance never even know that anything happened to them. They get an overnight stay in a plush suite along with several rides up and down the hall in a wheelchair.

If the cash patient had a voice (and until now they haven't), this would not be the case. They don't want us to have one either. After all, doctors are human, even though they don't act like it. I think some doctors have a deep-seated desire to hurt someone, and they can do it to a cash patient and get away with it.

When my girlfriend, Patty, arrived at the hospital to drive me home, Dr. "Pocahontas" told her, "You have to stay with him for twenty-four hours, because he could bleed to death. You cannot leave him. If he changes in any way, you must call me and bring him here right away."

Patty took me home and I fell asleep. When I woke up a little while later, she was gone. I was alone without a car and the nearest neighbor was a mile away. I started to walk to the nearest neighbor because I figured that was where Patty was. I was pissed! I didn't knock; I just walked right into the neighbor's house, ready to kill. After all, I've got Schering Plough's best answer to hepatitis C in my blood: interferon alfa-2b recombinant, Intron A.

Sure enough, there she was. She was "snorting" cocaine, a joint in one hand and a mug of some good hard liquor in the other. I could tell she was deciding which of the several young males surrounding her would be her next victim. I could see it in her eyes.

Driven by the wonder drug in my system, I was vicious. My look nearly killed her and a few innocent bystanders. I swear there are a few unfortunate people out there who probably had heart attacks and strokes that were induced by me while I was under the influence of interferon. After realizing the danger of being with an individual on interferon, and still having a desire to live long enough to corrupt a few more souls, Patty decided to drive me home.

I also destroyed everyone I knew. I called Patty's husband and told him I was having sex with his wife. I informed him that I had been having sex with her since their wedding day when he had passed out and she went looking for someone to abuse.

During the entire year of 1995, I actually completed two weeks of full doses and ten weeks of half doses. Interferon destroyed my brain. My left knee felt like it had a blowtorch on it for months. I almost crashed my truck on several occasions. I got sicker and sicker, until I swear I was almost dead. Yes, I'm convinced I was within hours of death.

Back in 1983, when I was working at Carol Merrill's restaurant, The Whale Watch, I could barely walk. As soon as Carol saw me, she insisted on taking me to see Dr. Ed Wagner, a Chiropractor and healer. He practiced in his own home, just around the corner from The Whale Watch.

For four years I could not stand up and walk like a normal person. I was taking numerous medications for this problem. Attempting to avoid surgery, I went to Dr. Wagner, who prescribed chiropractic manipulations and gave me extensive diet instructions.

After about three weeks of his treatment, I was walking just fine. Now after sixteen years, I rarely have back pain, something eleven surgeons told me could be relieved only by surgery.

Nearly every time over the last sixteen years when I left Dr. Wagner's office, I felt that something had happened that I didn't understand. So many times I walked down his driveway wondering what went on in there that caused me to feel so good.

When your spine is adjusted properly, your entire outlook, mood, attitude, and feelings change for the better. You feel good! I believe his type of treatment was beneficial to my triumph over hepatitis C.

I bought a computer and spent hours on the Internet searching for information about hepatitis C. I was astounded to discover how much was being done around the world for hepatitis C, with great results, but not in the U.S.

My neighbor, Jon Chann, tried for months to convince me that I should see Dr. John Finnegan, N.D. Finally I agreed. At the same time, I made an appointment with a hepatologist at Cedar Sinai Medical Center.

ON A QUEST – ROAD TRIP

About seventy-five miles north of Los Angeles, Patty had a burger fit. Malicious, ball-busting female, I should have left her at home. She had no less than fifteen burger fits between Los Angeles and San Jose. Anytime she saw a Burger King or an In & Out Burger, this woman would threaten to orgasm if I stopped.

The people out there on Highway 5 are different. They are like characters out of a 1950's horror movie like *Godzilla*. These people haven't been to college. They spend their lives aspiring to work pumping gas at the local truck stop. They've reached their goal, and it can be dangerous dealing with a person who has reached their goal, especially when they are half your age.

Between burgers, Patty drank from a gallon of milk mixed with two quarts of Kahlua that she had hidden in an

19

ice chest. That woman can suck down more liquor than any man I've ever known or heard of. Patty's gone now, dead I think. Although maybe she's living somewhere like Laguna Beach – and just millimeters from being institutionalized.

Patty was never any fun on a road trip. She believed she should only fly first class or ride in a limo. She considered this trip – five hundred miles in a Toyota truck – to be the low point of her miserable existence. However, we had a common destination. She was going to be the bridesmaid at Kathy and Chris' wedding in Saratoga on September 7, 1996, while I was hunting for the west coast distributor of live cell thymus, the main ingredient necessary to conquer hepatitis C. San Mateo was my destination. My quest: to convince the highest person in that company that I had to have thymus to survive.

I am a carpenter and could not afford to pay quadruple inflated prices for it. After all, we are talking about a very expensive cut of beef. This is not something regulated by the FDA.

We arrived in San Jose and checked into a hotel. Patty was not happy; there was no room service and no elevator; it was very primitive. She called the nearest liquor store, ordered everything that would fit on my credit card, and had it delivered. I went to sleep.

It was six a.m., September 5, 1996. I knew Ms. Patty wouldn't be awake until four p.m., so I went to San Mateo. Driving was so much easier when I didn't have a drunken lizard sharing the front seat with me.

I had called ahead and made an appointment with a Mr. Q. At our meeting he told me he was really sorry, but he had a contract to distribute this product only to health care practitioners.

I had anticipated his response, and I had a very real and sympathetic saga, which I delivered to him. I attempted to appeal to his human characteristics. He didn't have any. I got what I expected. Now it was back to hell, or at least to the gathering area for those headed there.

I dared not awaken the drunken lizard, for admiration of life was something still securely attached to my being. Slowly though, she awoke and floundered around for a long while. Then she decided that she deserved a dinner in a fine French Bistro.

When it came to spending someone else's money, Patty was very professional. She collected herself, examined the yellow pages, and called her friends in the wedding party. Her main objective was not to greet or say hello, but to get them to help her locate the most expensive, most elegant French restaurant within a sixty-mile radius. She was successful. She got directions, painted on her make-up, and off we went.

I felt like I was dying. I felt like there were maybe only a few hours of this life left. I had felt this way often during the past two years. Saratoga, with its quaint tree-lined streets, was a lovely place to die. I parked my truck, my lovely reliable Toyota truck. It always started and ran. If America made cars more like it, we'd still own Hawaii.

What happened next had to be told to me by Patty, because I do not remember it.

She said that I could not sit in the chair at dinner. I kept sliding down and passing out; my eyes were open. I ordered a half bottle of non-alcoholic wine. She told me that I could not remember anything. I had not had any drugs or alcohol for who knew how long. I did remember the outside of the building, the streets, and the trees. I also remembered the peace. The nearness of death and the peace it promised. I felt very sick almost all the time.

I didn't remember the food. She said it was good. We walked down the street while she smoked several cigarettes

21

before the ride home, as there was no smoking allowed in my truck. I was sick and couldn't understand why she was trying to get sick. This woman smoked every conscious moment and consumed any and all available alcohol or drugs. She generally felt miserable at least twenty-six days a month. All I was searching for was life. It was during times such as these that I was ashamed that I didn't spend more time attempting to be a doctor of anything, at least then my vocabulary would be such that I could express my true feelings more appropriately.

September 6th, the day before the wedding, was the first and only time I had been instructed by Patty to awaken her before dark. The wedding party had invited about thirty-five people in Saratoga to brunch. What a wonderful group of people they were. It's very rare to meet so many wonderful people all in one room.

The brunch was very casual, with plenty of champagne. You could have anything on the menu with no restrictions. This was truly a celebration. Even though I was practically comatose, I remember the grace, generosity, and celebration to which these people were dedicated. Before this, I'd only read about such an event.

That evening in Saratoga, we were at the finest restaurant in town, and we could have all the food we ever wanted. The father of the bride was a very happy man. Truly he was a great man by anointing his daughter, his future son-in-law, and all their friends with such a great event. There was an extraordinary feeling of well-being and friendship in the air that was felt by all.

I was very embarrassed to think that these wonderful people might wonder what was wrong with me. Yet, as sick as I was, I remember thinking that this event must be as good as going to heaven would be.

The next morning we were off to some former Senator's house for the final celebration. It was very nice, except that while dressing, Ms. Patty had a romp with her male counterpart in the ladies' bathroom. Not what one would expect from a traveling partner during what were most certainly his final days. Commitment was something with which the newly weds were adorned. However, Ms. Patty lacked it; in fact, she swore it would make her vomit.

There was another dinner after the wedding in a remote place on a large creek. It was a great setting. Patty had wandered off somewhere else. By now, many of the people in the wedding party had been introduced to me, and they began to ask, "What is wrong with you?" I told them I had a terminal disease, hepatitis C.

Most people think hepatitis C is something you get from drinking too much. Really, people don't have a clue.

The wedding was an exquisite, gracious three days of ceremonial bliss. The following morning the newlyweds took several of us out for a late brunch. This was the first time I'd paid an ATM fee of three dollars for a forty-dollar transaction! I was really slipping. My ability to function rationally was in an advanced stage of deterioration, a stage where you gravitate from here to the other side.

The wedding was a most joyous celebration of life. It reminded me of the story about Jesus and his first holy miracle of turning water to wine at the marriage in Canaan of Galilee. Kathy and Chris' wedding was the first wedding I've ever attended where the bride and groom maintained composure at all times.

Thank you Kathy and Chris for allowing me to share your blessed wedding with you, and may love be with you always. The time I spent with you and your family and friends was a turning point in my life. When I arrived at your house, I was so sick I could hardly walk and I felt like

23

I was near death. The love, kindness, and compassionate concern shown to me by you and everyone I met during the three days I spent with you gave me the determination to continue living and the strength and will to search for a cure for my life-threatening disease. I will never forget the date, September 7, 1996, the date you were joined.

I was on a quest to purchase the main item that leads to recovery: live cell thymus extracted from the thymus gland of calves.

HIGH-PRICED
PROFESSIONAL ADVICE

In 1996, I attended an appointment I had been waiting for, for over a year. This was partly because it took months to get in, but mostly because it took years to save enough money to pay for the appointment.

I drove anxiously down Pacific Coast Highway to Wilshire Boulevard, where I encountered massive quantities of lunchtime traffic that consisted of drivers from all classes of misfits frantically roaming the streets at lunch hour. I was angry, having traversed this town many years earlier and knowing somewhere in my brain that I knew exactly where I was and where I was going.

I thought I missed the turn. I was confused due to the toxins in my blood interfering with my brain function. I was sort of not all there and not in control. The minutes ticked off. I was angry, but steeped in high anticipation. I was elated at the prospects of attaining information from the doctor who was supposed to be the greatest possible source on the planet earth for information about the disease that was killing me.

Yes, here I was, after long anticipation, waiting to absorb every great morsel of healing news that would be entering my ears. I was ready to absorb all of the previously unknown, invigorating medical information that was about to be bestowed on me by the esteemed highest of the high: _-_ _ _-_ _ _ M.D., hepatologist of the Liver Transplant Program at Cedars Sinai Medical Center.

The waiting room was huge, larger than anything I'd ever seen. It was impeccably decorated. I only enjoyed the great magazine selections for a few short moments, and then I was whisked away into the chamber where, in only moments, I would meet the "Great Hepatologist."

_ _ _ _ B.S.N., R.N., the hepatology nurse, took my blood pressure. It was 178/140. She was sweet, very nice and gentle. Then the hepatologist entered.

He was about my age, seemed uptight, and asked questions for about an hour. He said these questions were very important.

He attempted to convince me that interferon was the only possible route to take.

Four or five times he said, "The one thing I dislike more than anything else is treating a patient who is intelligent and well read, and you are intelligent and well read."

He also told me there was nothing he could tell me to do or not to do; there was nothing I should or shouldn't eat; nor was there anything I should or should not take. He said that after my test results were back, he would call me and discuss them with me.

I ask him for his opinion regarding a high albumin count and its effects on the immune system. I explained to him what I had recently learned about albumin. He told me "That is the most ridiculous thing I have ever heard."

This visit cost me $788.00.

I went home and began redirecting my efforts toward finding a source for live cell thymus on the Internet.

"THE GREAT" HEPATITIS C RESEARCHER AND ELVIS

I had begun taking live cell thymus several months prior to my visit to the "Great Hepatologist," along with a regimen of other items, many of which I had never heard of before. John Finnegan, N.D., prescribed them for me.

The items consisted of things like Reishi mushrooms (real "shrooms," not a pill) and making teas two or three times a week that took me six hours to make. Fortunately, since then I have formulated different ways of making the teas so they take much less time.

I boiled milk thistle seed and made a tea from it too. No tea bags, no pills from a bottle, but real things from real plants. The preparation was time-consuming, but hey, this is my life. Modern medicine gave me all it had, and modern medicine failed!

I also took lipoic acid. My brother told me about a doctor he had heard on a radio show in Washington who treated hepatitis C with vitamin C injections combined with lipoic acid, a vitamin co-factor. My understanding is that lipoic acid is something that complements vitamin C in the body. I took lipoic acid plus two to three thymus capsules two or three times a day and many other new and interesting items, not vitamins, but food in pill form.

Soon I began to feel much better, especially on the days when I took the live cell thymus. At first I took it twice a week. Taking it caused me to feel completely normal, health-wise that is, so I began taking it more often, and then every other day.

About three weeks after my visit to the hepatologist, his terrific well-mannered and proper nurse (whose clothes I wanted to tear off and have wild sex with right there in the reception room) called me to inform me that most of the tests had to be redone. The liver panel was good and showed that the three indicators were three and four numbers above normal. This was a great reduction from my previous battery of blood-sucking, money-grabbing testing.

One year later, I was broke. I had exhausted all of my assets seeking out the secret, expensive health knowledge buried in catacombs. Now I began to understand why.

I made an appointment with the "Great Hepatologist"– UCLA's best hepatitis C research doctor. He was considered the number one researcher at the great, noble and respected UCLA Medical Center – a leader in the world today and a teaching institution that passes on the great tendencies of arrogance, those beliefs they're paid to find and make sure that not anything else is said.

I drove directly to the UCLA Medical Center, passing by the welfare office on Veterans Street, where two years earlier I tried to get some help with the expensive and deadly interferon. I was confused and disoriented as I paid my five dollars at the parking center, so I asked someone at the information center to direct my sickly being to the entrance of the digestive disease center. When I arrived there, I was whisked away into a hallway; my blood pressure was taken, and I was weighed on a scale in kilos. I had to translate the kilos into pounds, because the nurse could not read the chart. I was asked the usual questions: "What drugs do you take? Are you allergic to any drugs?" I listed my herb intake and she wrote herbs on my chart.

After waiting for about ten minutes, and having read and researched every item in the "vacuum," a beautiful student doctor came into the room. She was nice, and she asked the usual questions, such as: "Are your feces black? What kind of drugs do you use? Do you have multiple sex partners?" and "Are you a homosexual?"

As she was about to leave, she told me the "Big Chief" would be in soon, and oh yes, she needed to perform a prostate exam. She said, "Please pull down your pants." I thought, "Sure baby, how about a quickie while we're at it? Hepatitis C is not a sexually transmitted disease so let's go." She really laid on the grease. Truly she should specialize in prostrate examinations because her finger was so small, and she was really good at it.

After she was through, she left, and the hepatitis C research doctor entered the room. All I could think of was the grease that was soaking through my pants, because she had not given me any paper to clean with. After this was over, I was going to have to walk out of there, and people might think I went in my pants.

31

The doctor said a few words, nothing remarkable, and then sent me to the lab for blood work. In between, I was fleeced for $188.00, plus lab fees of $360.00, making a total of $548.

The blood work technicians seemed like students, and they were certainly from a different economic class than the workers at Cedars Medical Center. Mostly rich Israelis occupy Cedars, making it truly a safe place to be. UCLA is more like a school. Nobody there seemed completely confident, except for the hepatitis C research doctor, and he thought he knew it all.

The "blood sucking" technician ripped a hole in my arm, causing my deodorant to fail and perspiration to flow, all because she would not listen to me. Finally, after a near death experience, she got help. I was bandaged, treated for shock, and sent home.

A few months went by. Two days before each of my scheduled appointments, someone would call and leave a message. I would call back and change the appointment to a few weeks later, because I had no money. I've always had a hard time making it to doctors' appointments if I didn't have money to pay for them. Someday, I might need a good mechanic (i.e. doctor), and I wouldn't want to be denied one because I had failed to pay a previous bill.

On May 29th, I drove past Mezzaluna restaurant, briefly contemplating getting away with murder. I entered the medical center parking facility and someone working at the tollbooth asked me, "Have you been here before?" "Yes," I responded. Then she said, "You mean I don't have to give you a long dissertation about where you're going?" I thought, "Oh no, not unless you can elaborate on how to get to heaven."

I got on the wrong elevator with an older gentleman, and the elevator only stopped at the parking lot levels.

After much button pushing, we arrived right where we had started. He got excited and stayed right by my side, as if I were the Messiah. Finally, I escaped from him by sneaking past a wheelchair in another very crowded elevator.

I got off on the wrong floor; well anyway, the stairs were cool. The waiting room offered a day-old LA Times food section about Nepalese cactus, something I grew at my Rancho Loco in Malibu. When you cook them, they're really slimy, like okra.

I went down the hallway, where a young lady took my blood pressure. She said, "Let me have your arm." I said, "Where would you like it?" She wasn't sure how to respond. However, she knew how to read a kilo scale, and I went off to the same vacuum I had examined on my prior visit.

A young male Japanese doctor – a tall, confident and pleasant-mannered fellow – came right in and immediately began reviewing my blood test results. He said I was in perfect health and I should see a psychiatrist. I requested a look at my blood tests, and sure enough, they were perfect. They were not just perfect, but absolutely perfect, from top to bottom. He took my test results back, and said the Big Chief would be in soon.

Next I saw the great and all knowing hepatitis C research doctor who said, "Mr. Wright, you are well. You no longer have any sign of disease. We could not find any hepatitis C virus in your system. Your blood test numbers were perfect. I'm going to refer you to a psychiatrist."

"I guess my live cell thymus program worked. Pretty cool, huh?" I said,

His uneducated response was, "Some people think Elvis is still alive."

I tried to tell him about my two thousand dollar a month romance with the various herbs that had cured me, and he responded, "Some people believe Elvis is alive and has two heads. All that stuff is crap. It has absolutely no use whatsoever. Stop wasting your money on junk, and use some of it for a few visits to a good psychiatrist. You will feel three hundred percent better. He will give you a little pill that won't hurt your liver, and you won't believe how good you'll feel."

As cautiously as possible, I attempted to tell him more about my herbal intake. I felt it was necessary for him to understand that I had been healed from a terminal virus by using herbs, supplements, and foods. The virus that causes hepatitis C afflicts five to fifteen million Americans! Perhaps they too could benefit from my expensive research and discovery. After all, he was a research doctor, a specialist in interferon research. Needless to say, he refused to even listen to the facts I offered him.

I had documents from several doctors over a six-year period showing my liver numbers from various labs before, during, and after interferon. I had documented proof that after interferon (and before taking herbal remedies), I still had hepatitis C, and my numbers had begun to rise.

After a year and a half of taking herbal remedies that are available to everyone on the planet, I was well. No hepatitis C was detectable in my system, and the American medical machine does not want you to know about it.

I was paying this man cash for his time, and all he did was make jokes about Elvis. I was thoroughly appalled.

Now I clearly saw why modern medicine could not cure the common cold: because no one funds this kind of research! They just fund things that suppress symptoms. If they cured disease, the money machine would stop. Sounds unbelievable, doesn't it? I have been in the "chamber of the gods" and they only have allegiance to their pharmaceutical funders, rather than to the patient and his or her welfare.

We live in a society where doctors deny reality and only adhere to their own agendas. Though this is difficult to believe, I experienced it time and again as I dealt with hepatitis C.

During the hepatitis C research doctor's dissertation including Elvis jokes, he claimed herb use was not documented and therefore invalid. The reason research of this type isn't happening is because people like him refuse to consider it. The pharmaceutical companies have a vested interest in suppressing natural remedies because they can't make any money from patenting them. Somehow, it seems to me that a man in this doctor's position could be saving thousands, and even millions, of patients from years of immeasurable suffering and prolonged agonizing deaths, if what worked on me was made widely available to others. He was in a position to help this happen, and he dismissed it with jokes about Elvis.

What I learned from my long, painful, and frustrating journey was that the efforts of one naturopathic doctor in Malibu and one chiropractor – two professions that are looked upon with skepticism – and my extensive research into natural alternatives had worked for me and literally saved my life.

MEDIA HYPE: THE POLITICAL MACHINE

The cumulative number of AIDS cases reported to CDC through June 2001 was 793,026. The total number of adult and adolescent cases was 784,032, with 649,186 cases in males and 134,845 cases in females. During the same time period, 8994 cases were reported in children under age 13.

The total number of deaths from AIDS was 457,667, including 452,111 adults and adolescents, 5,168 children under age 15, and 388 persons whose age at death was unknown. (CDC Semiannual *HIV/AIDS Surveillance Report.* These numbers are based on AIDS cases reported to CDC through June 2001.)

The Center for Disease Control and Prevention states that 4,000,000 Americans are infected with hepatitis C and at least 2.7 million of them have chronic infections. The

Los Angles Times reports that at least one half million people in California have hepatitis C and at least 41% of the prison population is infected. The misery, suffering, fear, and expense to people with hepatitis C are experienced by millions of Americans, while AIDS is only affecting a small portion in comparison. While the number of AIDS related deaths has dropped significantly over the last few years, the number of deaths from hepatitis is expected to triple over the next ten years.

Over ninety percent of the people with hepatitis C caught their destiny from a blood transfusion, other hospital procedures, or dental work. I noticed that during the annual hepatitis C conference in Chicago, the media hype emphasized that hepatitis C is a sexually transmitted disease (STD). Hepatitis C is not an STD!

It's true that doctors like to say this during their conferences, but they do not mention the fact that most of us got this "great reward" in doctors' offices and hospitals.

As a result of the way we contracted hepatitis C, we are a random section of the populace, not a clear and distinct voting block. Since politicians want the support of a distinct voting block, those with AIDS benefit, and those with hepatitis C do not.

In the United States, hepatitis C doesn't have the organized group effort that it has in Canada. It's truly random. You are in a traffic accident, go to the hospital, receive a blood transfusion, and die from hepatitis C. You want some perky "tits," so you go to a plastic surgeon, who transforms your "droopers" into "mammoth mammaries," and you pay with your life.

There are those who received the reward of hepatitis C from needles by injecting their good times, not knowing that they were playing Russian roulette with an as yet unknown disease. Hepatitis C was only discovered in 1989, a mere twelve years ago.

As most Americans have heard, hepatitis C is a celebrity disease. Mickey Mantle, David Crosby, Naomi Judd, Pamela Anderson, and Larry Hagman are just a few of the celebrities who have suffered from hepatitis C and its complications.

As a result of the public outcry about giving preference to celebrities, the National Transplant Association changed its rules. All hepatitis C patients are now considered third state recipients. That means if you have hepatitis C, you are less likely to receive a liver than someone with a non-contagious infection or life-threatening condition.

The Association's reasoning is that the disease that is carried in the person's blood will also infect the new liver, and they will eventually die anyway – unless they read my book. A person in a traffic accident who needs a new liver, and wasn't drunk while driving, will get a liver before a person with hepatitis C.

If you were in a traffic accident that caused you to get hepatitis, because you went to the hospital and got a tainted transfusion, where lies the morality of the events that generated the new guidelines?

Those of you who are reading this book probably won't need a new liver. I have not researched this much because I could never afford a liver transplant. The government won't give me Medi-Cal coverage, so I know I will never have a new liver. Still, the bureaucrats and the doctors responsible for the current guidelines have their heads in the clouds.

I want the whole world to know about the horrendous injustices resulting from the voting blocks reported by the media. I want the world to understand that the search for a cure for disease appears to be more aggressive when it is based on the greed of politicians responsible only to their voting blocks. Also, doctors hide from their responsibility in spreading hepatitis C in the United States.

When the whole picture is examined, it causes one to look down and sadly shake his or her head, while the special interest groups, politicians, and doctors are saluting the flag.

In fifteen Asian countries, experiments are being conducted that are producing excellent results in curing hepatitis C. The products used in these experiments cannot even be purchased in the United States.

PATS REPORT:
I'D BE DEAD BY NOW

In 1997, a letter from the Hepatitis Foundation International (HFI) found its way to the "stomach" of my baseball bat-beaten mailbox. Enclosed was a form with a space for my phone number. If I signed and returned it to 30 Sunrise Terrace, Cedar Grove, CA, I could be put on something called the PATS Report. This report contains a list of names and phone numbers of other unfortunates with the same infirmity as I had.

The list arrived. It was on yellow paper with black ink. It had first names, phone numbers, cities, and hepatitis interest - a clever way to discern who had B or C or both. After scanning through the list, I decided to call some of the people living in the cities closest to me.

41

"Bill" from Canoga Park was my first call. He answered and was right up front with me. He said he had done a lot of speed and figured he got hepatitis from dirty needles. He didn't know for sure. He told me that his son also was infected with the C virus. His words about the doctors that he and his son have supported financially intersected with my pool of disgust, the depth of which amazed even me. It was October 18, 1998, and the bastards still didn't get it. Bill told me that his doctor told him not to worry as long as it didn't bother him.

Why does advice such as this cost hundreds of thousands of dollars? It's for education resulting in the capital letters accompanying a person's name, letters that lend distinguishing results such as Dr., M.D. or Ph.D.

For me, college was some drink, lots of sex, and running naked across the college campus. It was also fast sports cars along with a degree of ethical behavior that resulted in what I'm putting down on paper in this book. Truly, I wish that I had spent more serious effort at almost everything in life.

The silent killer is working on Bill and his son. A simple change in diet and a few herbs would make a vast difference in the progression of their illness.

Bill had a fax machine, so I faxed him a copy of my "bad blood" test results, a copy of my liver biopsy, and the results of two other blood tests. One is dated September 22, 1998, and the other is dated April 10, 1997; both tests are perfect and show no RNA viral infection of hepatitis C. I included a copy of my herb list and diet.

A while later Bill called back. He was filled with enthusiasm and wanted to know where to get the items I was taking. I shared all of my information with him. It was a list of things that cost me thousands of dollars to compile. I did this just so he could get well.

Herein lies my need to tell the whole world about how I recovered. While the program I followed may not cure everyone, I believe the research I reviewed for this book supports the belief that it should work on most humans the way it worked on me. Good luck Bill and please remain on my program.

Next I talked to "Mary" from Melview:

"I'm tired. I can't remember what my doctors said. I've taken to the Lord. God will deal with it. Never would I take something, unless my doctor told me to."

She asked, "Are you a doctor?"

"No," I replied.

She said, "Well, you should be ashamed of yourself for pretending you can cure something. Shame on you."

I couldn't help this woman.

If she read her *Bible*, she would find out that in the Old Testament God said he had provided all the herbs needed to cure all the infirmities that would affect man.

She did mention that heavy donations to her church were sure to save her; certainly I don't disagree with giving to your church. I know God can (and sometimes does) heal.

When I had cancer, I went to church every Sunday. I attended prayer meetings and was baptized in a nearby swimming pool. My name was printed alongside Michael Landon's in the church paper each week asking for prayer.

One fine day, the preacher preached a whole sermon about how badly he needed a clear plastic pulpit to stand behind. It would signify power and bring strength to our small gathering of born-again believers.

It was a time when I was very sick, and I was taken in by his request. I asked the preacher how much it would cost and promptly wrote a check for five hundred dollars.

A few months later that fine, clear plastic pulpit arrived and that preacher was standing behind it with his fly down!

I was in the front row and was so embarrassed. After about two hours he finally discovered his fly was down and then spent two more hours disciplining the congregation for allowing him to carry on without telling him.

A few months later that preacher bought a washing machine for a tribe of nuns in Africa, a place where they had no laundry detergent, hot water, or even electricity.

Shortly after that, he ran off to South America with a good-looking girl from the choir and the church bank account. He left his wife, his friends, and everything else, except the money. I guess he needed the money to carry out the Lord's work?

Please don't get me wrong here, I love God and I know he created me. I could not be here, if not for him. A strange thought just occurred to me. How many doctors do you know who believe in God?

Basically, in my pursuit to help the people listed on the yellow PATS Report, and the other people with hepatitis C that I've meet, I've encountered three distinct types of responses: the interested, the disinterested, and most of all, the "I wouldn't do anything unless my doctor told me to do it." I'd be dead by now if I had followed that uneducated, uninformed train of thought. The response, "I wouldn't do anything unless my doctor told me to do it," came through in the testimony of almost all of the people on the PATS Report list.

Now, seven years later, after speaking with over 40,000 individuals infected with the hepatitis C virus, I still find these three general types. The difference is that two-thirds of these people have used interferons and the various combo treatments only to have them fail. They are now looking for a healthier life. Most of the others I communicate with are people who have done some research and discovered that there is not much good written

44

or said about "The Drug Company Cure." Except, of course, what the drug companies write or pay to have written. People who do research try alternatives first.

Most of the people who contact me tell me the same story: "My doctor said 'herbs, diet, and nutrition do nothing for hepatitis C.'" Their doctors don't know how to cure hepatitis C; and, of course, they haven't bothered to do any other research in order to save the lives of their patients. This still baffles me. Was I a mutant? Perhaps I've missed some important dose of civilized behavior along the way. I am reminded of a movie, *Soylent Green*, where people just walked right into this huge machine that turned them into food. Only Charlton Heston rebelled and exposed what was going on. Was Timmy Leary right? Did that acid trip I took when I was twenty really open my mind?

Please read *Hepatitis C Free: Alternative Medicine vs. The Drug Industry: THE PEOPLE SPEAK*. Get a copy and give it to your doctor as a present. We need to help educate them. After all, someone needs to. Ninety-nine percent of what the average doctor knows about hepatitis C is from a flyer he read that was distributed by a drug company or from a seminar he attended put on by a drug company.

10

THE LETTER:
DOES ANYBODY REALLY CARE?

For those of you who believe my brain is permanently damaged – which at this time I have no quarrel with – I bring you more evidence of the used-car-salesman mentality of the key people at the pinnacle of the pillar of crap called "The Fight Against Hepatitis C." I bring you their lack of interest and their blatant disregard for the facts about which they are supposed to inquire.

I have included a portion from the newsletter, *Alert*, published by the Hepatitis Foundation International (HFI). This organization constantly sends me material requesting cash donations to support its yacht and Rolls Royce payments. The following is from the issue dated Fall 1998:

47

HFI'S CEO Serves on NIH Alternative Medicine Planning Committee

Thelma King Thiel, Chair and CEO of HFI has been invited to serve on the complementary and Alternative Medicine (CAM) Planning Committee at the National Institute of Health "I'm pleased to be representing patients and HFI in this effort to evaluate the safety and effectiveness of complementary and alternative treatments for hepatitis and other chronic liver disease," said Mrs. Thiel. "The fact that Congress has appropriated an additional $50 million to the Office of Alternative Medicine is very encouraging."

The CAM Planning Committee has been formed to assess the current knowledge of complementary and alternative medicine for chronic liver disease, focusing on the availability of scientific evidence for efficacy and safety; to identify and prioritize research needs that will fully define the efficacy and safety of CAM for liver diseases; and to form a consensus on the state-of-the-art of CAM for liver disease. The committee hopes to disseminate the consensus to both the medical and lay communities through (a) the publication of the conference proceedings and an executive summary, and (b) publication of lay informational materials disseminated through NJDDK clearinghouse and lay foundations.

Reading this newsletter excerpt was one of the highlights of my existence. I was healthy, and I tested hepatitis C non-detected. Immediately I called Thelma King Thiel and spoke with her secretary. She informed me that her boss would love to speak with me about my ordeal and cure; however, her boss was currently on a conference call and would call me back as soon as she finished.

During my conversation with the secretary, I told her about my battle and eventual cure and that UCLA had declared me hepatitis C free. She asked me to fax some material regarding my illness so Ms. Thiel could have a look, as they were very interested. She gave me the fax number and within minutes I faxed the following documents to her:

To: Thelma King Thiel
From: Lloyd Wright

I read last night that you were invited to serve on the CAM planning committee. I was infected with hepatitis C in 1979 from a blood transfusion. It was finally diagnosed in 1994. I cured it with alternative medicine.

I would like to discuss this with you, because I believe it could help many people and most doctors. Those I've told about my program do not take me seriously.

Thank You.

Lloyd's Liver Biopsy Report:

Surgeon: D. MD
Date of Surgery: 12/16/94
Date Accessioned: 12/16/94
Blocks: 1
Recuts:
Stains:

Specimen (s):
Liver biopsy
OR Consultation:
Gross Description:

The specimen is labeled "Lloyd Wright, UTSD liver Biopsy." It consists of two thread-like pieces of soft pink-white tissue measuring 0.7 cm in length and 1.5 cm. In length and averaging 0.1 cm. In diameter or less. The tissue has a stripped appearance. TE-1. RLR: do

Diagnosis, including microscopic examination:

Chronic hepatitis consistent with hepatitis C; UTSD liver biopsy (see microscopic description and Comment).

a. The sections show hepatitis tissue with moderate to marked chronic lymphocyte inflammation that is predominantly periportal. Focally lymphocytes percolate out into the hepatic lobules in the sinusoids. There is mild to focally moderate steatosis with predominantly large droplet fatty change. In some of the portal areas, the bile ducts appear attenuated by the inflammatory process. The features are consistent with hepatitis C infection. Definitive piecemeal necrosis is not seen. Mallory's hyaline is not seen. Special stains for iron reveal minimal focal positive staining involving hepatocytes. Special stains for connective tissue reveal a mild to moderate periportal fibrosis with a few portal areas showing tendrils of bridging fibrosis. No regenerative nodules of cirrhosis are seen.

Comment: The Tissue block will be sent for hepatic iron analysis at MLN. Results will be forwarded as soon as they are received.

Completion Date: 12/20/94
RLR:sg

CAL Clinical Laboratories			
Patient: Wright, Lloyd			
Sex: M Age: 40			
Lab # 4783255			

Date of Specimen: 01/30/91   Time Reported: 5:54 AM

Hematology	Results	Units	Ref. Range
WBC	6.38	Thous/CMM	4.30-11.0
RBC	5.18	M/CMM	4.7-6.1
HGB	16.1	GM %	14-18
HCT	46.7	%	42-52
MCV	90.2	CU Micron	77-102
MCH	31.1	M MCGMS	27-32
MCHC	34.5	%	32-36
Platelet Count	273	Thous/CMM	130-400
Neut	67.3	%	50-75
Lymphs	26.8	%	20-40
Monos	4.1	%	0-10
Eos	1.6	%	0-5
Baso	.2	%	0-3

Biochemistry – A			
ALKP'tase, Total	115	MU/ML	30-115
LDH Total	234	MU/ML	100-250
AST	**210**	MU/ML	1-41
ALT	**245**	MU/ML	0-45
GGTP	**215**	MU/ML	0-65
Total Protein Serum	8.5	GM/DL	6.0-8.5
Albumin	5.1	GM/DL	3.0-5.5
Globulin, Total	3.4	GM/DL	1.9-3.5
A/G Ration, Chemical	1.5	Ratio	1.0-2.2
Bilirubin, Total	.5	MG/DL	0-1.5
Bilirubin, Direct	.1	MG/DL	0-.4
Bilirubin, Indirect	.4	MG/DL	0-1.2

DISPLAY/PRINT   STANDARD DISPLAY   THU 05/29/97 0852
RESULTS   COLLECTED   PAGE 01 BY
                                    LAST 4 MONTHS   LM@LDK

DISPLAY/PRINT RESULTS	STANDARD DISPLAY COLLECTED LAST 4 MONTHS	THRU 05/29/97 0852 PAGE 01 BY LM@LDK
PATIENT ID 219-29-02 1	PATIENT NAME WRIGHT, LLOYD	SEX AGE UNIT/S RM/BED TEMP M 47 LOCATION

PTEST NAME 04/10/97 1430	F RESULTS (COLLECTION TIME)	UNITS 1527 (IN LAB TIME)	REF RANGE
CHEMISTRY PANEL			
CHEMISTRY PANEL COMMENT	PROFILE PERFORMED		
SODIUM, PANEL	139	mmol/L	136-146
POTASSIUM, PANEL	4.1	mmol/L	3.6-5.0
CHLORIDE, PANEL	102	mmol/L	97-110
CO2 CONTENT, PANEL	28	mmol/L	25-32
GLUCOSE, PANEL	89	mg/dL	65-110
CREATININE, PANEL	0.9	mg/dL	0.5-1.2
UREA NITROGEN, PANEL	12	mg/dL	8-20
TOTAL PROTEIN, PANEL	7.6	g/dL	6.0-8.0
ALBUMIN, PROTEIN	4.7	g/dL	3.7-4.8
PHOSPHORUS, PANEL	3.4	mg/dL	2.6-4.2
BILIRUBIN, TOTAL, PANEL	0.7	mg/dL	0.3-1.2

TEST NAME	F RESULT	UNITS	REF RANGE
04/10/97 1430 (COLLECTION TIME)	04/10/97 CONT'D.	1527	(IN LAB TIME)
CHEMISTRY PANEL			
ALKALINE PHOSPHATASE, PANEL	86	U/L	35-110
AST (SSGT), PANEL	23	U/L	5-50
ALT (SGPT), PANEL	12	U/L	5-50
CHOLESTEROL, PANEL	239	mg/dL	0-240
CALCIUM, PANEL	9.8	mg/dL	8.4-10.0
TSH	0.9	mIU/L	0.3-4.7

END OF REPORT

Radiation Center Date of Specimen: Time Reported: 09/22/98 4:30 AM		Patient: Wright, Lloyd Sex: M Age: 48 Spec. No. 44291763	
Test Name	**Results**	**Ref. Range**	**Units**
Basic Metabolic Panel			
Glucose	99	65-110	MG/DL
Sodium	145	135-148	ME/QL
Potassium	4	3.5-5.5	ME/QL
Chloride	102	95-107	ME/QL
CO2	26	22-34	ME/QL
BUN	19	6-25	MG/DL
Creatinine	.9	.5-1.4	MG/DL
BUN/Creatinine	21.1	10-28	Ratio
Albumin	4.5	4.1-5.4	G/DL
Bilirubin, Total	.4	.1-1.5	MG/DL
Bilirubin, Direct	.1	0-.3	MG/DL
ALK Phos, Total	**49**	30-125	U/L
AST	**21**	1-45	U/L
ALT	**14**	1-45	U/L
CBC w/Diff			
WBC	5.5	4-11	X10*3/CUM
RBC	4.54	4.2-5.5	X10*6/CUM
Hemoglobin	14.9	13-17	GraMs./DL
Hematocrit	42.9	38-50	%
MCV	94	82-97	Cubic Mic.
MCH	32.8	27-34	PicograMs.
MCHC	34.7	32-36	%
RDW	11.6	11.5-15.2	%
Platelet Count	175	150-400	XFL
MPV	8.4	5.2-11.1	0*3/CUM
Neutrophils	61	50-70	%
Lymphocytes	23	15-50	%
Monocytes	13	0-10	%
Eosinophils	2	0-5	%
Basophils	1	0-5	%

Let's go over this again. Thelma King Thiel, Chair and CEO of Hepatitis Foundation International, was invited to serve on the Complimentary and Alternative Medicine (CAM) Planning Committee at the National Institute of Health. She commented:

> I'm pleased to be <u>representing patients</u> and HFI in this effort to evaluate the safety and <u>effectiveness</u> of complimentary and alternative treatments for hepatitis. The fact that Congress has appropriated an additional $50 million to the office of Alternative medicine is very encouraging. The CAM planning committee has been formed to assess <u>knowledge</u> of complimentary and alternative medicine for chronic liver diseases. (1) (Emphasis added.)

Considering what you've just read, think about this: I faxed Ms. Thiel a brief letter stating I was cured from chronic hepatitis C. I included a copy of my liver biopsy dated 12/16/94 as proof of the severity of my disease. The biopsy was performed at Los Robles Hospital in Thousand Oaks, California. I also included a copy of one blood test from 1/30/91, showing my AST (SGOT) Panel at 210 when it should have been between 1 and 41. My ALT (SGPT) Panel was at 245, which should have been between 0 and 45, and my GGTP at 215, which should have been in the range of 0-65. I sent a copy of the results of this test because it was easily accessible, and it showed a long period of time between tests, indicating I'd been infected for many years.

I also faxed to her a copy of the results of my blood test taken on 4/10/97 at UCLA. This test showed AST (SGOT) Panel at 23, normal range between 5-40 and ALT (SGPT) Panel at 12, normal range between 5-50. These results were better than perfect. They indicated that my liver functions were better than normal for a person of my age with my history. It was, in a word, phenomenal. It was not a miracle, but the results of dedicated study and practice of what I had learned.

Further, I faxed Ms. Thiel a copy of the results of a blood test taken 9/22/98, showing AST (SGOT) at 21, normal range 1-45 and ALT (SGPT) at 14, normal range 1-45. These test results were selected because they were my most recent and showed that even as I continued with my naughty habits, I continued to stay well after years had passed. These tests proved that I was cured of hepatitis C. I've read about other cases, and I know first hand that this did not happen to most of the people who survived treatment with interferon.

This material should arouse the interests of anyone, especially a foundation determined to help find a solution for this disease. However, it didn't seem to interest Ms. Thiel. I thought it would because of her new position. Please absorb her letter to me dated December 30, 1998, on the following page. Read it two or three times, and then think about your fifty million in tax money that went to support "Alternative Medicine." Think about your health. If you have hepatitis C, wouldn't you want to know about someone who actually recovered and how they did it?

HEPATITIS FOUNDATION INTERNATIONAL

December 30, 1998

Mr. Lloyd Wright
Malibu, CA 90265

Dear Mr. Wright:

Thank you for writing. I'm delighted that you are in good shape.

Fortunately, recent research reports indicate that many people with biopsies like yours will not advance to serious liver disease, but will remain healthy carriers. This is very encouraging news.

Good luck and stay well.

Sincerely,

Thelma King Thiel
Chairman and CEO

Hopefully, you've digested the fact that people like Ms. Thiel, who are in high places, just don't give a damn.

Here is another example that shows how hepatitis C is being handled in a fashion that defies belief:

Naomi Judd, often referred to as "The Queen of Country Music" is a truly fascinating personality. The American Liver Foundation (ALF) sent out thousands of copies of letters written by Naomi, wherein she described her feelings when she was diagnosed with hepatitis C and how hepatitis C had changed her life. She described her daily awareness of the "spirit, mind, body connection," and how she has dedicated her life to finding a cure for hepatitis and other liver diseases.

By the end of the first page you are undoubtedly about to sob, but by page two, the tears begin to flow as Naomi relates to you how her first course of treatment with interferon in 1990 didn't work. She writes:

> I was so sick...and so scared. I thought I was going to die. In 1996 I started a second course of interferon treatment, and when this was finished one year later, my doctor told me that the virus could no longer be found in my blood. I was so happy. I still can't stop thanking God. However, many people do not respond to therapy, so I am dedicating my life to finding a cure because there is so much more we need to know... and do. (2)

I wondered what "and do" means? She knows the cure? Could it be that the Liver Foundation didn't want her to say it?

Naomi goes on for about five more paragraphs hyping interferon, the research of the American Liver Foundation, hoping for more treatment options, and begging you to send your hard-earned money to this callous organization.

She pleads, "Please join me in accepting... responsibility and with your generous contribution, creating a 'Campaign of Hope' that will support the essential work of the American Liver Foundation."

Well Naomi Judd, "National Honorary Spokesperson," you are a most elegant and remarkable person. However, as I see it, you speak with forked tongue, or perhaps hepatitis C caused a lapse in your memory?

Let's go back to the January 1998, issue of *Alternative Medicine Digest*:

> Naomi spent the next six years looking into a range of alternative medicines. A program of nutritional and herbal supplements strengthened her immune system and lent support to her beleaguered liver. She takes...." (2)

The article goes on to describe many of the same things I did: vitamins, milk thistle, thymus, and glandular extract from calves. "Naomi's liver enzyme levels, which had gone up again after the interferon cycle ended, dropped to within the normal range, after she added the thymus glandulars to her program." (2)

It's remarkable what you can find out there if you've got the money and the energy to find it. Money alone won't do it. From what I read in the *Alternative Medicine Digest* article, it seems that Naomi and I have had very similar experiences.

I am very pleased that she is well, but it does bother me that she sells interferon with what appears to be great enthusiasm and leaves out the genuine pieces of healing news for you to find elsewhere. But the ALF probably just pays her to say what they want her to say, not necessarily the whole truth.

Hopefully Naomi will go back and demand that the ALF allow her to tell the entire story. She owes it to everyone who has this dreaded disease.

Unfortunately, this type of dirt and corruption persists throughout the entire spectrum – wherever there is a dollar to be made.

11

HEPATITIS C, PANCREAS AND CANCER

After publishing the first edition of this book, I began documenting a plethora of cases where hepatitis C carriers also had blood sugar disorders, including type II diabetes; most of these people had also used interferons. I further researched other sources such as *Hepatology, A Textbook of Liver Disease* (3), and discovered that it has long been contemplated that the pancreas is an additional breeding ground for viral hepatitis. In this book, authors David Zakim, M.D. and Thomas D. Boyer, M.D. discuss the relationship between viral hepatitis and pancreatic dysfunction and that pancreatitis has been found on autopsy in viral hepatitis cases:

61

It has been known for more than 40 years that viral hepatitis can co-exist with acute pancreatitis. Most instances of overt pancreatitis have occurred in association with fulminant hepatitis, and hence the most reliable figures come from autopsy examinations. Necropsy studies have defined pancreatic involvement in 12 to 40 percent of patients with fatal hepatitis, with pathologic changes ranging from slight pancreatic edema to severe hemorrhagic pancreatitis. It has been suggested that the pancreatic necrosis may be triggered by disseminate intravascular coagulation. Of note is the accumulating evidence that the pancreas might represent an important nonhepatic site of viral hepatitis. A disturbance in pancreatic endocrine function in patients with hepatitis has also been reported. One group of investigators observed abnormal glucose tolerance in 50 percent of patients with viral hepatitis. The diabetes was attributed to direct invasion of the pancreas by the hepatitis virus.

Additionally, after interviewing many doctors at different conventions and Universities where I have spoken, I ascertained that it is not unusual for viral hepatitis carriers to die from pancreatic cancer. The latter data was discovered and circulated when hepatitis C was first labeled as Non A/Non B.

Within a year of publication of *Triumph Over Hepatitis C*, I learned that the unfortunate guinea pigs of modern medicine who signed onto Peg-Intron trials were developing high rates of type II diabetes. As I was constantly craving sugar, I became my own first case study using pancreatic enzymes. After I began taking Pancreas Organic Glandular, my sugar cravings began to diminish.

Within the past year, a client informed me that she had developed diabetes so I suggested she try Natcell Pancreas and she agreed. After only a few weeks, she called to say that her doctor had reported that her tests had improved. She subsequently used Natcell Pancreas for three months until her diabetes was controlled. Since then, several of my clients have developed type II diabetes from the use of Peg-Intron and Ribavirin. Additionally, clients call and tell me that their mother, father, or friend has diabetes. Many have tried the Pancreas Organic Glandular for blood sugar problems, and all have reported great results. (Blood tests on file.)

It is critical to note that over ninety years ago, Dr. John Beard discovered that pancreatic enzymes are a great cancer treatment, as evidenced in the following excerpt from an ABC news report:

JOHN MCKENZIE, ABC NEWS

More than 90 years ago John Beard, a Scottish scientist at the University of Edinburgh, documented cases of cancer patients successfully treated with pancreatic enzymes. Normally pancreatic enzymes produced in the body help digest food, but when taken as supplements on an empty stomach, they appear to be absorbed into the blood stream and attack cancer cells throughout the body. Dr. Nicholas Gonzales has now treated more than 400 patients with a variety of advanced cancers.

Mort Schneider's body was riddled with tumors.

MORT SCHNEIDER:

The surgeon told my wife that I really didn't have very long to live, possibly a few months.

JOHN MCKENZIE:

That was nine years ago. Today, he's still taking the enzyme supplements. As for the cancer, those tumors, four in his liver and one in the pancreas, have all disappeared. Even more impressive to the scientific community was the small pilot study Gonzalez published last year: Eleven patients with advanced pancreatic cancer, the most deadly form of cancer, where the average survival is only about six months, were put on enzyme therapy. These patients lasted an average of 17 months, almost three times longer.

If left untreated, many hepatitis C carriers will develop cancer. More significantly, those with hepatitis C who use interferons are at greater risk of developing a wide range of cancers. Thyroid cancer, primary liver cancer and cervical cancer are among the highest reported. Remember, I am still early on this investigation, and cancers can take years to develop.

Kidney failure, while being a complication of hepatitis C, is more common in people who have used interferons.

Currently I am researching glandular therapies for the reversal of kidney problems and the results are promising.

Cancer is something we all want to avoid. Current therapies are barbaric and lack proper support for our immune system. Interferon is a cancer drug. It lowers the white blood cell and platelet counts. This allows bacteria, infection, and cancers to enter the system and start their destruction of the body. Put simply, interferons put the immune system to sleep.

The following is part of the warning label on Schering Plough Corporation's interferon packaging.

> **WARNING:** Alpha interferons, including PEG-INTRON, cause or aggravate fatal or life-threatening neuropsychiatric, auto-immune, ischemic and infectious disorders. Patients should be monitored closely with periodic clinical and laboratory evaluations. Patients with persistently severe or worsening signs or symptoms of these conditions should be withdrawn from therapy. In many, but not all cases, these disorders resolve after stopping PEG-INTRON therapies.

If you still decide to use interferons, please consider using an immune system boosting program so you can avoid suffering later because you put your immune system to sleep with these toxic treatments.

Many retired medical doctors, who now promote alternative treatments, have informed me that prior to the 1989 discovery of HCV, there were many deaths reported from primary liver cancer in people who had a hepatitis Non A/Non B diagnosis, yet the connection between the two was never made.

Recently, the media has reported that primary liver cancer diagnosed in the victims of hepatitis C has jumped from 10% to 40% after 20-30 years from contraction. Having been prevalent in every member of my family and having survived my own bouts with this disease, cancer continues to alarm me. I have been told that due to the type and quantity of radiation I received, I am now 9 times more likely to develop another cancer than the average American. One out of every two average Americans develops cancer at some point in his or her life. Just three years ago it was 1 out of 3 and ten years ago, it was one person in 4. These are alarming statistics.

In conclusion, I implore you not to use interferons. I hope I can help you prolong your time on earth and minimize your suffering by showing you what does work, what worked for me, and what is working for so many others. If you have hepatitis C, DO NOT USE INTERFERONS. Ask yourself this: Why are there no long-term studies on interferons? The reason is because people who use interferons are either dead or still sick.

The pancreas is an important organ in the human body because it produces substances required to digest nutrients and controls blood sugar levels. The name 'pancreas' has a Greek origin "pan," which means "all" and "creas" which means "flesh." Protect and support your pancreas.

We can help prevent cancers by using a few well-known preventative measures. These are alternative prevention measures referred to in many books, but not well-known in the "modern medicine era."

Prevention is the most important and reliable cancer-fighting tool that exists today.

Foremost among the preventative measures is to maintain a strong and healthy immune system. This can be accomplished by practicing the remedy in this book, maintaining a diet that ensures the optimal intake of immune system enhancing nutrients, and decreasing your intake of immune system suppressing foods. Living a life free from constant emotional or mental distress is very important, as is avoiding carcinogenic toxins, geopathic zones and harmful electromagnetic fields in your home and work environment.

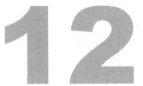

THE DARK AGES:
IS THIS REALLY PROGRESS?

Ethics, morality, they no longer exist. It's as if we were strung out on a long acid trip enhanced with a pound of good Afghani hash and a few buttons of peyote. Then, there appeared before us a giant eraser, and we wiped ourselves clean.

It's all about image. Image is all there is, whether it's your own, corporations, the great renowned learning institutions, or the corner store. It's just image. There is no substance. Doctors are a prime example of this illusion. They even want you to imagine yourself well. An article in the Fall 1998 issue of *Hepatitis Alert*, titled "Placebos & Positive Beliefs Help Healing" states, "An enthusiastic

69

physician who provides encouragement that the treatment will work provides hope and optimism to patients." (4)

This statement indicates to me that if I have a good doctor and he tells me that the poison known as INTERFERON ALFA-2B RECOMBINANT will cure me, and I believe him, then I will be just fine. What is this, the "Dark Ages?"

We are the first people inhabiting the earth who feed our most precious meat source a strict diet of chicken manure and "40 billion pounds a year of slaughterhouse wastes such as blood, bone, and viscera, as well as the remains of millions of euthanized cats and dogs passed along by veterinarians and animal shelters." (5) This means that the remains of America's pets are being used as cattle food and have been for years. Cattle are also fed ROAD KILLS, dehydrated food garbage, fats emptied from restaurant fryers and grease traps, cement kiln dust, newsprint, cardboard, hog manure, and yes, we even feed our cows human sewage sludge. (5) Truly, most of us are literally full of manure.

Our prestigious learning institutions and great medical facilities have even dumped their cadavers, mixed with toxic waste, into the Santa Monica Bay.

These cadavers were the remains of the great and noble people who donated their bodies to science in order to further the study of all things that plague humans. In return, they were promised a proper burial.

In the name of the almighty dollar, The University of California at Los Angeles (UCLA), and no doubt other institutions, burned these cadavers slightly and then tossed the remains in the bay.

An LA Times article dated February 23, 1994 documented this practice:

Without admitting guilt, UCLA has agreed to pay $49,500 and strengthen its medical waste practices to settle charges that it violated the law in disposing of human remains at its medical school. UCLA and the State Department of Health Services said that they were happy with the agreement, which stems from an October 1993 incident in which the skipper of a burial-at-sea service accidentally broke open a box of ashes that UCLA wanted dumped into the Santa Monica Bay. The box contained cremated remains of cadavers used by UCLA Medical School, but also contained pieces of glass and surgical equipment. (6)

In this article, the skipper of the boat and one state investigator said that hair was also found on some of the remains and rubber stoppers were still in some bottles,

...indicating the possibility of a low temperature in the incinerator that burned the remains. (6)

In the settlement, UCLA agreed to close its on-campus crematorium and send all cadavers used by its medical school off campus for disposal and burial. A Department of Health Services Investigator (named McGurk) indicated that the fact that UCLA was an institution supported by students and taxpayer funding figured into the monetary settlement. What we didn't read, but must know, is that there was no doubt a huge profit stuck in the pockets of those few individuals at the medical school who carried out these illegal, evil deeds. Surely there were large bills for

71

proper burial and big costs for proper cremation. The manner in which the entire incident just disappeared indicates big payoffs. UCLA teaches ethics in more places than its classrooms.

What we as a society have become is, in the strictest sense, phenomenal. I've been trying to tell people about the unethical operations of many renowned institutions for years. People think I'm nuts when I tell them that the American cows' diet is chicken manure. I've seen those seventy-five foot high mounds of mixed rations on cattle ranches in many places around the U.S. We are in DENIAL!

On February 23, 1994, the U.S. News and World Report Online stated:

> Toxic heavy metal: arsenic, lead, cadmium, and mercury can collect in organs and tissues of cattle. Effects on humans who eat tainted beef are uncertain. (7)

However, what we eat has a lot to do with why we die. One in two of us will be greeted with cancer, and eating meat from cows that are fed a chicken manure diet doesn't help us. Who is stupid here? We think we can't afford to feed ourselves, or the world, so we have lapsed into a state that cannot continue. A great decline will surely take place, and we will be forced to adjust our behavior.

Since the sixties, I have been listening to individuals tell me red meat is bad. Many people express all sorts of unusual effects from eating cows, including feeling dirty. I believe that many of us are sensitive to red meat because of what the host animal was fed.

If you concur that the development of these unethical practices is in the name of saving money, then it becomes easy to see that we cannot afford to feed ourselves. Our attempts to feed ourselves have become futile.

Our farmers have been over-farming the same land for hundreds of years. In most cases, farmers are only replacing three chemicals in the earth: nitrogen, potash, and phosphate. This has been practiced throughout the last half of the 20th century. There are hundreds of known trace minerals, nutrients, salts, and probably unknown quantities of other elements that have been depleted from our soils and these elements are no longer in our food.

The government tells us we are living longer, healthier lives. They say we eat better than any humans who lived before us, and that our medical technology is the best in the world.

I haven't heard any news recently about the righteous. We can't say God in a public school, and Jesus Christ has become a swear word. People claim they're spiritual, when they only gather a little here and a little there, and then combine these "littles" in their minds to equal spiritual.

Our lives are overburdened with getting here and getting there. We've developed "always being late" as socially proper. I hate to suggest this, but I'm going to: we have developed into a "herd" culture, and I wonder if it has anything to do with what we eat.

As I see it, most of us are overweight, fixated on plastic surgery in a vain effort to impress the opposite sex, and dedicated to "Self."

I ponder how many of the people who have elected to have unnecessary plastic surgery will die early because of the tainted blood they received from transfusions or the unsanitary instruments that were used in the operating room.

Things as common as having your children's teeth straightened or cavities filled have no doubt created many cases of hepatitis C.

Hepatitis C is a deadly virus that is able to *hide* inside the liver cells. Because of this, the virus is able to survive the immune system's attack. Macrophages and Kupffer cells are activated in the liver by the immune system to release chemicals to destroy the virus. The liver cells are exposed and the liver becomes the unintended victim. Cell death and cirrhosis follow.

Our government, various liver disease agencies, and the majority of doctors want us to believe that there is no specific group of people who have hepatitis C, because they don't want the power of a group that might demand answers. They want us to believe it is just random people who are unfortunate enough to have received a tainted blood transfusion. Blood transfusions are by far the number one culprit, but intravenous drug users and gays and lesbians have a higher incident of hepatitis C than the general population.

Dr. Teresa Wright, Chief of Gastroenterology at the San Francisco VA Medical Center says, "Hepatitis C is the one nobody talks about." Dr. Wright claims that the hepatitis C virus goes into hiding for years while it quietly works on the liver. "Eventually the result is cirrhosis or liver failure, which is fatal without a transplant!" Dr. Wright also noted that ten percent of the patients admitted to the VA Medical Center, for whatever reason, carry hepatitis C in their blood. At least eighty percent of all those who contract the virus develop a chronic infection. During the past few years, the Veterans Administration released figures indicating that 65% of Vietnam era veterans are infected with hepatitis C. (8)

There are many intelligent people out there who can think, in contrast to the vacuum of the Federal Drug Administration (FDA) and its whole group of followers. It seems that the FDA, as well as the majority of the doctors practicing "Modern Medicine," feels they need to create cures. They have concocted a whole new line of chemistry with really great side effects. It brings you to a near-death experience, trying to kill whatever it is that is killing you, so you can survive in a seriously impaired state.

It would be wrong of me to simply stop here with the feeding and eating of cows. You may, if you believe what you've been told, decide to eat fish instead and think you'll be safer. You decide you are going to board a fishing vessel and go out and catch your own. Let the light be shed. I have a neighbor named Andy who is a salmon fisherman. In recent years the number of salmon has plummeted, and their size is approximately one third smaller than it was just a few years ago.

Salmon swim up stream to spawn, and there are many fish hatcheries up many streams. Agencies sponsored by the U.S. government are attempting to increase the number and size of this slippery little fish by raising them in hatcheries. Because of the use of all sorts of growth hormones, these salmon have lost much of their color. Now they're feeding them dye as well, in order to give these mutants the color of the lost race.

Occurrences of human interference are not simply limited to salmon. This sort of human tampering is being done all over the U.S. Human interference with nature produces terrible unknown consequences.

Recently newsrooms were flooded with reports of genetically modified corn making its way into a certain brand of taco shells. The modified corn was created to kill a certain weevil that infests cornfields. The idea was that if science could cause the corn to kill the weevil, the farmer could use less insecticide. It turns out the modified corn makes humans sick, so they feed it to cows. Then we eat the cows. A loophole in the law, which is occurring as I write, allows corn producers and processors to turn tens of thousands of tons of genetically modified corn into corn syrup and train car loads of it are arriving daily at the three major vitamin C producers in the U.S. Yes, they are making vitamin C out of genetically modified corn!

You might also be surprised to learn that all of the soybeans grown in the U.S. are genetically modified, unless they are labeled "organic."

"Why?" you may ask. The answer is to cut down on cost of labor in farming and harvesting. Genetic modification was implemented to avoid manual labor weed removal.

The problem: Roundup is increasingly being used and traces of it can be detected in almost all of the soy products that are not labeled "organic."

Another problem: The air moves; it's called wind. Pollen does not stay in genetically modified fields; it is carried everywhere by the wind.

The biggest problem, however, is that Roundup is in part being manufactured from recycled Agent Orange, the defoliant used in the Vietnam "Police Action" to defoliate Vietnam so we could see the enemy. Ask any Vietnam veteran about the effects of Agent Orange.

I cannot say this is simply crazy. This is outright mass stupidity. The "Almighty Buck" is the prime motivator. Human health, and the future of the human race, is ignored and forgotten for the sake of immediate corporate profit.

Ever fly over Los Angeles and land at LAX? Don't look down! If you do, you will see miles and miles of structures created by people for people, tens of thousands of them.

The humans living in all these structures use toilets several times each and every day. All this human waste, along with a multitude of other toxic chemicals, is pumped into the sea. Not just Los Angeles, but along almost every coast in the world, and guess what those little fish eat? Makes you sick, doesn't it?

Back when "King" Richard Nixon reigned, his "think tank" determined that the number one problem facing the world was not nuclear war, but overpopulation.

In America, it appears we are attempting to deal with overpopulation on several fronts: raising animals fed with waste products for human consumption, condoning abortion, and allowing people to die who could be saved. The FDA doesn't want to hear anything about alternative solutions such as the healing power of herbs.

> And God said, 'Behold I have given you every herb bearing seed, which is upon the face of all the earth, and every tree in which is the fruit of a tree yielding seed; to you it shall be for meat.' Genesis 2:29 *King James Bible*

News Flash! February 12, 1999, 10:30 a.m. KNX news radio reports: "The FDA has approved radiation treatment of meat to kill bacteria." Isn't that what we used to kill the Japanese in WWII? The FDA probably does not know that radiation isn't selective about what it kills. It will probably turn meat into a glowing fiber.

Several years after this, Americans will no longer be reproducing, cattle farmers will be broke, and cattle experts will no longer exist.

You can imagine the headlines of the future:

Meat-Packing Company Over-amps Meat!

300,000 Die as a Result of Radiation Poisoning!

As a result of what happened in New York on September 11, 2001, the U.S. Postal Service has begun radiating the mail to kill anthrax. We can only imagine what this radiation is doing to what we send through the mail.

I am in a quandary. This process of radiation is not news to me. It just simply never occurred anywhere in my brain that the group of fools who are doing this could possibly be that stupid. It reminds me of those commercials on the *Ed Sullivan Show*, "BETTER LIVING THROUGH CHEMISTRY." Although we are still cleaning up the DDT in our environment, generations from now we will probably still be suffering from its effects.

What is even more preposterous is that the poor unfortunate and misguided don't believe cows eat chicken manure and they don't care if they do. They don't care because they are not convinced that this could be true of "their" meat. The possible consequences of this apathy are beyond imagination. Future headlines for many years to come surely will reflect on such decisions as "bombarding" our meat with radiation or feeding cows waste.

The reason these issues are so important is that part of almost everything you eat, drink, smoke, snort, or inject goes into or through your liver. It is the largest organ in your body, and it performs over twelve hundred different functions.

If your liver is sick, the very first thing you must do is make a decision: do I consume things that will surely destroy my liver, or do I only allow things into my liver that will not jeopardize its condition and will nourish it and help it rebuild?

78

Obviously, any creature – human or otherwise – will pay a price if it eats food that is not intended for it – or if it eats any food that was nourished on food not intended for *it*. The representations produced by laboratory analyses of the content of food are misleading in determining the needs of living organisms in the real world. (9)

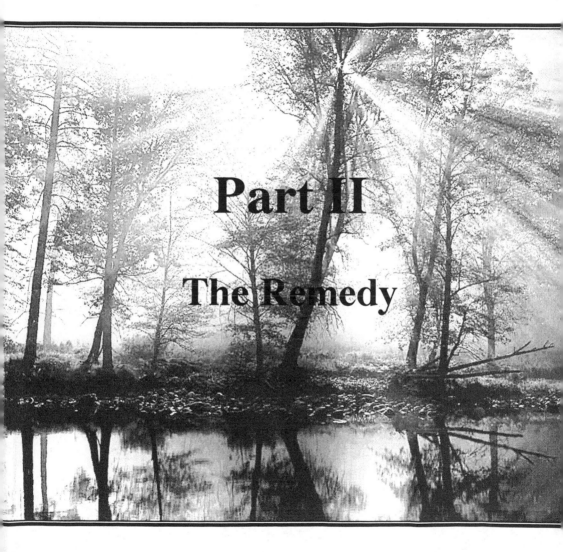

Part II

The Remedy

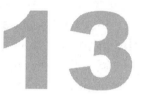

WELCOME TO THE REMEDY: THE ALTERNATIVE MEDICINE SOLUTION THAT SAVED MY LIFE

In essence, no two people react exactly the same way to any medicine, herb, or group of herbs. You need to be intuitive and follow your inner direction. Develop sensitivity toward your being and experience the response. Keep uppermost in your mind that you can, and must, take responsibility for your health. You can adjust your life and health better than anyone else can.

The quality of herbs and supplements depends on how they are grown and processed, which will then determine how much benefit your body will receive from them.

It is not the herb or supplement that heals you alone, it is your immune system that monitors and protects your body. You must fuel your immune system with what it needs to do the job.

Liver cells degenerate in hepatitis C and B in a similar fashion. The damage done to the liver is actually caused by the reaction of the immune system to the virus.

The immune system sends special immune cells equipped with powerful chemicals to the liver. The virus is able to <u>hide</u> inside the liver cells. Because of this, the virus is able to survive the attack by the immune cells.

Macrophages and Kupffer cells are sent to the liver by the immune system to release chemicals that destroy the virus. The liver cells are exposed and become the unintended victim. Cirrhosis and cell death follow.

Peptides are the tiniest of protein molecules. They are found in live cell thymus and live cell liver, as well as other live cell glandulars. Peptide growth factors actually communicate with the other cells in an organ. To simplify, they actually orchestrate the attack by the immune system. They communicate with each other and alter their own behavior. These peptides actually convey information inside their animal host.

Mucopolysaccharides are found in properly prepared aloe vera, reishi mushrooms, and shark cartilage.

Dr. John Finnegan, states:

> These 'leaders' (polysaccharides), the beta-glucomannans have a unique penetrating action which acts as a biological vehicle drawing nutrients through the tissues and cells of the body. They actually penetrate the cell wall and become incorporated into the cell wall, carrying with them the body's own immune cell fighting mechanism.

This process takes time and requires dedication. It is necessary to help support the liver function through proper diet, the elimination of toxic material, boosting the immune system through proper nutrition, and protecting the liver during this process by consuming the herbs, foods, and supplements discussed in this book.

Please keep in mind, I used very few supplements for three years after I was declared non-detected by UCLA on April 10, 1997. In 2000, my book began to sell, my research increased, and now that I am able to afford these supplements, I continue to take them daily as the PCR test is not refined enough to determine if the virus is completely gone. If it is lying dormant in my system, I want to keep it dormant. As of October 5, 2001, my PCR is still non-detected, ALT 13, AST 17.

The supplements I recommend to people with hepatitis C who wish to improve their health are discussed in the following chapters.

HOW TO PREPARE THE TEAS

If possible, use distilled water in the following:

HYSSOP – energizes and cleans.
Bring 2 quarts water to a boil. Remove from heat and add 1 cup of hyssop. Cover and brew for 1 hour. Pour through strainer into container. Refrigerate after cooling and enjoy!

MILK THISTLE – regenerates your liver and can help reverse cirrhosis.
Bring 2 quarts of water to a boil. Add ½ cup milk thistle seeds. Simmer for 1 hours, adding water as needed. Pour through a strainer into a container. Add water to seeds and run again through the strainer and into the container. Cool, refrigerate and enjoy!

REISHI MUSHROOMS – helps produce body's own natural interferon.
Begin with one medium size mushroom in two quarts of water and simmer in a glass container for six hours. Then, dilute by fifty percent and drink one-half cup twice daily, between meals. Be careful, because this mushroom can "amp" you easily. If you feel your liver swelling, drink less. It took me a while to get up to two cups a day.
The pre-sliced mushroom slices are easy to make tea with. Soak approximately 25 mushroom slices overnight in water, simmer for 45 minutes, and strain and enjoy. Remember that you can only brew Reishi mushrooms in a glass container.

LICORICE ROOT – a great anti-viral!
Bring 2 quarts of water to a full boil and remove from heat. Add ¾ cup of licorice root. Brew for 1 hour. Pour through

strainer into container. Refrigerate after cooling and enjoy!

DANDELION ROOT – removes toxins from your blood and reduces brain fog.
Rinse ½ cup of dandelion root in a strainer. Use a 2-quart pan with lid. Fill with 2 quarts water and bring to boil. Add ½ cup of the rinsed dandelion root. Remove from heat and brew for 1 hour. Pour through a strainer into a container. Keep a large supply in the refrigerator and drink as iced tea.

CAT'S CLAW – a world-class herb with the power to arrest and reverse deep-seated pathology.
Make a tea from the inner bark. Bring 2 quarts water to a boil. Add 1 cup shredded bark. Simmer for 15 minutes. Let brew for 1 hour. Strain and enjoy! Warning: may cause drowsiness.

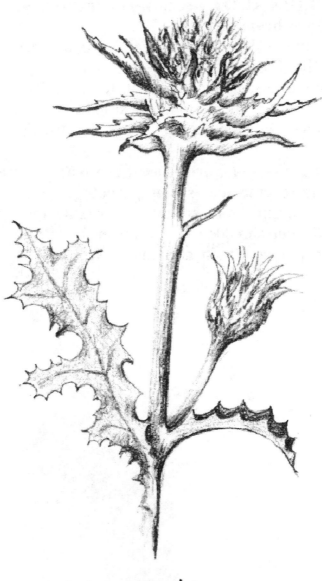

Milk Thistle

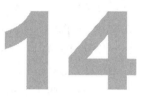

MILK THISTLE:
ANCIENT BLESSING

After I learned about milk thistle, I began taking this remarkable, ancient remedy immediately and never stopped. You can acquire it in most health food stores, and it is offered in a variety of forms. Some formulas combine it with artichoke leaves, dandelion root extract, licorice, and other herbs.

I use the organic seeds, simmer them for two hours, and then drink the tea iced. It is also important to take at least 1000 mg. of milk thistle per day in capsule form, in addition to the tea, as silymarin is not water-soluble. There are other active ingredients in milk thistle that are important, but unfortunately most of them are eliminated from the processed capsule form. This is why I recommend taking both the tea and the capsules. I've reviewed many articles and studies on milk thistle and hope that some of them will find their way to all those liver doctors who told me there was nothing I could do or take to help my liver regenerate.

For centuries, dating back to Roman and Greek civilizations, milk thistle has been used as an antidote for poisoning, including snakebites. Silymarin, which is derived from milk thistle, is considered medicine's most important antidote to poisoning by the mushroom toxins a-amintin and phalloidin.

Cited as one of the oldest known herbal medicines, milk thistle is part of the daisy family, and it is also a relative of the common garden thistle and the tasty artichoke. In Roman times, Pliny the Elder, a noted naturalist, described the medicinal uses of milk thistle, indicating this prickly medicine was excellent for carrying off bile.

Jean Rohrer comments:

> There has been recent clinical research, especially in Germany, which has brought the use of this multifunctional plant to front row prominence in the treatment of liver toxicity. Indeed, milk thistle is considered supreme in healing chronic or acute liver damage, virtually regardless of cause, as well as protecting the liver against many toxins and pollutants.
>
> First, silymarin stabilizes and strengthens liver cell walls, stopping toxins from entering. It acts by inducing formation of liver cell proteins, which are incorporated into the cell walls, making them stronger and more resistant to toxins.

Second, by increasing the rate of protein synthesis, silymarin enhances regeneration of liver cells.

Third, are the antioxidants and free-radical scavenging abilities of this marvelous weed. As if these impressive effects weren't sufficient, the fourth mechanism silymarin gets involved in is the enzyme and catalytic activity of the liver. It inhibits production of the enzymes that produce substances damaging to the liver, while at the same time preventing the depletion of glutathione on liver cells, a substance that mediates cell metabolism.

Clinically, milk thistle causes significant reversal of symptoms of both acute and chronic liver problems from viral hepatitis to cirrhosis. (10)

During my treatment I took:

Two 400 mg. milk thistle capsules three times per day. I also drank one quart of milk thistle tea per day.

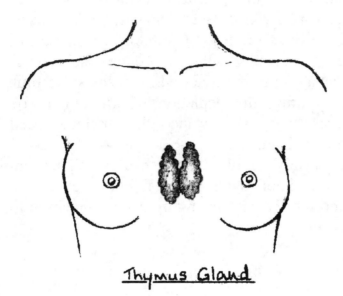

Thymus Gland

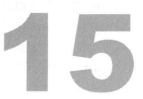

THYMUS:
THE FOUNTAIN OF YOUTH

The Thymus Gland is a small gland in the upper chest. It weighs 1/3 - 1/2 half ounce at birth, and reaches its peak weight of about 17 ounces at puberty. Thereafter, under the influence of many factors, including adrenal and sex hormones, the active thymus gland cells begin to die off, with much of the thymus gland tissue being gradually replaced by fat and connective tissue.

Much of the healthy thymus gland structure typically atrophies by age 20, and the decline accelerates throughout life thereafter. As immunologist Keith Kelly notes: "The involution (shrinkage) of the thymus gland is one of the cardinal bio-markers of aging." In the past 40 years, science has discovered that the thymus gland is the key regulator of immunity.

Collectively, thymus gland hormones have been shown, in human, animal and in vitro studies, to have a broad range of action, well beyond merely maturing and differentiating T cells. These hormones can prevent the tissue wasting that occurs with thymus gland removal or severe thymus gland atrophy, and promote healthy weight gain in disease states- such as AIDS – where catabolic body wasting is typical. The thymus gland hormones can reduce autoimmune reactions, clinically and experimentally, such as occur in rheumatoid arthritis.

Thymus gland hormones also prevent the bone marrow injury and subsequent reduction in white and red blood cell production, frequently produced by X-ray or chemotherapy cancer treatment.

As cellular physiologist Dennis Fahy has noted:

> If you restore immune function, your ability to make DNA, to have normal cell division, to have normal insulin sensitivity, to have normal thyroid levels and other things, such as normal population of certain molecules in the brain that change with age, all these things are restored by an improvement in the immune system.

Since thymus gland hormones are secreted by the very thymus gland cells that "shrivel up" and waste away due to aging, stress, disease, radiation and malnutrition, etc., the drop in thymus gland hormone activity with aging should hardly be surprising.

Although it is not well known, even to most alternative/ anti-aging medicine devotees, there is a large body of published, human clinical research supporting the use of oral thymus gland extracts. They have been used in a broad range of conditions, ranging from cancer treatment, to rheumatoid arthritis, to various allergy and asthma conditions, to recurrent respiratory infections and hepatitis. (11)

These studies have generally shown thymus gland extracts to be extremely non-toxic and side effect free, with few contraindications for use.

The main block to the acceptance of the efficacy of oral thymus gland extracts is the erroneous yet widespread belief that all proteins and peptides taken orally, as food or supplements, are 100% digested to individual amino acids before absorption, from the intestine into the body.

If this were true, then indeed orally administered thymus gland peptide hormone extracts would be broken down completely during digestion, becoming merely very expensive, low dose amino acid supplements, with no more immune activity than (for example) a few hundred milligrams of ground beef protein. Yet it has been known since the 1970's that significant quantities of various proteins, such as gliadin from wheat, milk casein, Ferritin, hemoglobin and milk immunoglobins routinely survive digestion and enter the body – and even the brain – intact.

The pioneering research of W.A. Hemmings and Ziovdrov and others had repeatedly demonstrated this by the late 1970's in a wide variety of experiments using many different proteins. (12, 33)

In the 1997 textbook *Oxidology*, Bradford and Allen even explain the mechanism of how this occurs. It is based on a cellular process called "pinocytosis." (44)

The thymus gland creates the T-4 "helper" white blood cells that perform their specialized job in the human body of locating invaders such as viruses, bacteria, or abnormal cells. The thymus gland also sends out the T-8 "killer" white blood cells to find invaders and destroy them.

People with advanced liver pathology will feel better after practicing the recommendations in this book. However, they may not completely reverse the path of the hepatitis C virus unless they incorporate the most aggressive treatment that delivers the best possible results: **NatCell™ frozen thymus extract.**

Enough cannot be said about live peptide thymus extract, which **feeds the immune system what it needs to kill the hepatitis C virus**. There are many forms of thymus: pills, liquid, natural, and artificial. These different products range from worthless to terrific.

I attribute most of the successful eradication of hepatitis C from my body as a direct result of consuming several thousand dollars of this product in eighteen months. Keep in mind that I had to pay as much as $600 a box to obtain thymus extract from doctors. I provide this same item for less than $140. I took one frozen vial every other day. I thawed it in my hand, poured one half vial under my tongue, and held it for five minutes, and repeat. If I could afford it, I would take it the rest of my life. If Cortez had found the fountain of youth, this could have been how he felt.

I advise against taking cheaper products. One example is Thymic Protein A, a product listed in *Health and Healing*, March 1997 (15). I took this product post-healing, and I did not notice the jolt or feeling of well-being associated with the natural form. I question whether or not Thymic Protein A is effective, as it contains only one of the seven main properties of the thymus gland.

Be warned, some of these products will not dissolve in water, even after an entire month. These pass through you completely and into the toilet. If you have hepatitis C, you need NatCell™ thymus extract!

Thymic hormones and their downstream cell products (such as interleukins and interferons) control all of the phases of maturation, development, antigen commitment, proliferation and cytotoxic activity of the various T cells. Thymic hormones also stimulate non-specific phagocytic and cytotoxic cells to respond against foreign or "non-self" antigens.

Liver diseases, including chronic hepatitis and primary biliary cirrhosis, have been successfully treated by thymus extract. Results of a study using 102 patients with chronic hepatitis and primary biliary cirrhosis showed an increase in T lymphocytes, increased functional activity of mononuclear cells (increased chemotaxis and inhibition), and decreased immunoglobulin counts. All of these indicators signify an increased competence, which favors controlling the immunoinflammatory process in the liver and a normalization of the clinical manifestation of the disease leading to a favorable outcome. (16)

These results are important not only for successful treatment of a very difficult disease, which frequently has an unfavorable outcome, but also for the implications for treatment of hepatitis produced by other causes. Viruses, fungi, or mycobacteria (tuberculosis) cause many of the inflammatory conditions of the liver. (17) Cellular immunity is the chief defense against these agents. Successful treatment using thymus extract suggests many exciting possibilities for treatment of the presently untreatable ailments of the liver using immunomodulating substances such as thymus extracts.

During my treatment I took:

One vial of Natcell Thymus on an empty stomach every other day for 18 months. I also took two 500 mg. thymus organic capsules three times per day.

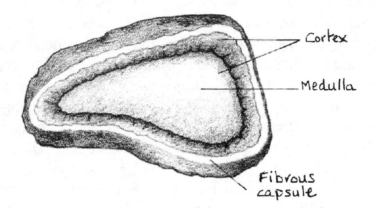

cross section of the Adrenal Gland

16

HEPATITIS C AND THE ADRENAL GLAND

The adrenal glands were first described in humans in 1563 by the Italian physiologist Bartolomeo Eustachio. Thomas Addison published the first studies on their functions only in 1855. The adrenal gland is extremely important in the fight against hepatitis C. Long-term stress, disease, chemotherapy and radiation therapy, including the use of interferons, can cause the medulla and the cortex to come apart. It is during this time that disease begins to spread.

Not surprisingly, "modern medicine" seems to have completely forgotten about the support of the adrenal gland while practicing barbaric life-threatening experimentation on humans through the use of Peg Intron.

The range of stressors to which individuals react is

broad: Physical exhaustion, demanding deadlines, infections, prolonged exposure to intense cold or heat, radiation therapy, chemotherapy, and major surgery all cause extreme pressure on the outer covering of adrenal glands due to discharge of high levels of hormones. These hormones, which are intended to help us survive stress, do so at a cost; they lower the immune system efficiency and body resistance leading to organ damage.

In order to support their adrenal glands, victims of hepatitis C should take adrenal gland concentrate, freeze-dried adrenal cortex, or best of all, but a bit expensive, Natcell Adrenal supplements. The adrenal gland aids the liver in regenerating new cells. (See Yale School of Medicine Study.)

Early research on T lymphocytes (defined as thymus-dependent cells, hence the designation "T"), shows that they express an immunoglobin-like two-chain antigen receptor (the TCR.) These cells are key components of adaptive immunity, express very diverse receptors, and are capable of enormous clonal expansion in response to an antigenic challenge. The relative expansion of specific T lymphocytes is part of the mechanism whereby a faster, more effective memory response is delivered on the second encounter with an antigen.

The liver displays extraordinary powers of regeneration after injury, but the mechanism underlying this capacity is not well understood. Minagawa et al. report that the regeneration of the liver after partial hepatectomy is accompanied by a large increase in the numbers of T-cell receptor-intermediate, mainly NK-like T cells. Further, they report that this increase is dependent on signaling through adrenergic receptors, because the beta-blocker (propranolol) and the alpha-blocker (phentolamine) inhibit the accumulation of these T cells. Minagawa et al. argue that adrenergic signals promote the recruitment of T cells. These two cell types may therefore be reciprocally regulated." (18)

Working in conjunction with the adrenal gland, the liver displays extraordinary powers of regeneration after injury and during and after viral attack. An article published by Yale Medical School entitled, "Do Natural T Cells Promote Liver Regeneration," emphasizes the importance of natural killer cells (T) cells in the regeneration of the liver. (19) Adrenergic Signals promote the recruitment of natural T Cells." Both Alpha and beta cells may be reciprocally regulated. What this means is that the adrenal gland and some of its functions are extremely important for liver cell regeneration. As evidenced by this article, the adrenal gland is still "not well understood," but one thing is certain, a healthy adrenal gland aids in the recovery from hepatitis.

Both hepatitis C and cancer patients can improve their health by taking Natcell Adrenal, which is a live peptide and they will notice a difference in their lives. Adrenal gland supplements can help the adrenal gland rebuild itself and also improve liver function.

During my treatment I took:

Two 300 mg. adrenal organic capsules per day.
I suggest taking Natcell Adrenal, one vial per week (optional).

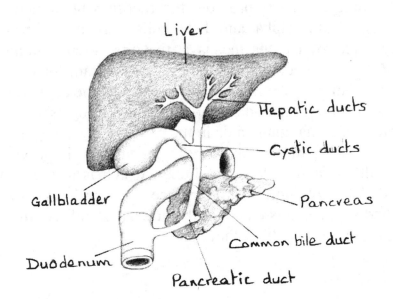

Liver

Hepatic ducts

Cystic ducts

Pancreas

Gallbladder

Common bile duct

Duodenum

Pancreatic duct

17

BOVINE LIVER EXTRACTS: PEPTIDE GROWTH FACTORS

Viral hepatitis is a fairly common systemic disease that is marked by hepatic cell destruction, necrosis, and autolysis, all of which lead to anorexia, jaundice, and hepatomegaly. More than 70,000 cases of the illness are reported annually in the United States. Today, five types of viral hepatitis are recognized:

- *Type A* (infectious or short-incubation hepatitis). The incidence of hepatitis A is rising among homosexuals and those persons with an immunosuppression related to an infection with the human immunodeficiency virus (HIV). The ingestion of seafood from polluted waters can cause it. People who are infected with hepatitis C, who also contract hepatitis A are in serious trouble. Recent statistics indicate a 40% fatality rate within 48 hours. The survivors are usually very sick for up to 6 months. Your doctor may recommend hepatitis A vaccine. Keep in mind that taking the vaccine will raise your hepatitis C viral load for a while.

• *Type B* (serum or long-incubation hepatitis). Also increasing among HIV-positive individuals, hepatitis B accounts for up to 10 percent of post-transfusion viral hepatitis cases in the United States. It is also transmitted by human secretions and by feces, such as during intimate sexual contact, and from the transfer of viruses into food prepared by infected restaurant workers.

• *Type C* (undetermined as to specific organism type). This disease organism is mostly acquired by blood transfusion from asymptomatic donors. Of all the hepatitis viral diseases, type C hepatitis is on the fastest rise among Americans. Hepatitis C is the most common reason for liver transplants in the U.S. today, and it is causing an alarming increase of primary liver cancer.

• *Type D* is found most frequently as a complication of acute or chronic hepatitis B, because this type D virus requires the hepatitis B organism's double-shelled surface antigen to replicate.

• *Type E* (formerly grouped with type C under the name *type non-A, non-B* hepatitis) primarily occurs among people recently returned from an endemic

104

area such as India, Africa, Asia, or Central America. Of the five viral hepatitis diseases, hepatitis B and hepatitis C are most dangerous because they have a high risk of developing into liver cancer.

Defining Live Cell Liver Peptide Growth Factors

From the Department of Pathology and Laboratory Medicine at Brown University in Providence, Rhode Island, U.S.A., three investigating pathologists, Drs. N. Fausto, A.D. Laird, and E.M. Webber, advise: "During liver regeneration, quiescent hepatocytes (liver cells) undergo one or two rounds of replication and then return to a non-proliferative state. Growth factors regulate this process by providing both stimulatory and inhibitory signals for cell proliferation." (20)

The idea of intrinsic hepatic growth control factors produced by animal and human liver cells has been stated in published reports, which date back to approximately forty-six years ago. (21-25) Much of this early research was conducted on rats and dogs, but currently clinical investigations among both healthy human volunteers and really sick people have taken place. (26)

Comprised of the tiniest of protein molecules, which biochemists and physiologists call *peptides,* these growth factors are of an exceedingly low molecular weight (30,000 Da), which yield two or more amino acids on hydrolysis. The Dalton with a symbol of D or Da, also called an *atomic mass unit,* is equivalent to 1.657 X 10 (24) gm. Peptide growth factors form by loss of water from the NH2 and COOH molecular groups of adjacent amino acids and are additionally referred to in biochemistry as di-, tri-, tetra-, etc. peptides, depending on the number of amino acids in the molecule. Thus, peptides make up the constituent parts of proteins. Examples of those several dozen peptides from the human liver and other organs which often give birth to growth factors are: hepatocyte growth factor (HGF), epidermal growth factor (EGF), transforming growth factor-beta (TGF-beta), and dozens more. (27-30)

According to which of the various scientific disciplines is being queried, different names exist for peptide growth factors. Historically, for instance, cell biologists have called members of their identified growth factor-type set of molecules "growth factors;" immunologists have named their growth factor-types "interleukins," "lymphokines," or "cytokines;" while hematologists have used the growth factor-type descriptive term "colony stimulating factors" (CSF). However, the present generally delineating nomenclature of "growth factors" has been and is now widely used throughout the world's scientific literature.

The term "growth factor" is now used consistently among almost every scientific and medical discipline, because in almost every case it reflects the context of the original discovery or isolation of any peptide. Since essentially all of these many molecules are multifunctional, it's not easy to conceive unique new names for them that would be entirely satisfactory; almost all of them are "panregulins," that is they react as universal regulators of the particular organ from which they derive. As you'll learn below, for the animal and human body, peptide growth factors are actually physiological symbols for the transfer of signals – a kind of language of biological regulation. (31-32)

Peptides often promote cell growth, but they also can inhibit it; moreover, they regulate many critical cellular functions, such as in the control of cell differentiation and other processes, which have little to do with growth itself. All peptide growth factors act in sets. To understand their actions, one must always consider the biological context in which they act.

Peptide growth factors provide an essential means for a cell to communicate with its immediate environment. They ensure that there is a proper local homeostatic balance between the numerous cells that comprise a tissue or organ. Since a cell must adjust its behavior to changes in its environment, the cell needs mechanisms to provide this adaptation. Therefore, the tissue cells, either singularly or collectively, use sets of peptide growth factors as signaling molecules to communicate with each other and to alter their own behavior to respond appropriately to their biological context.

The most important peptide growth factors of the liver's hepatocytes have been identified as a collection of hormones called "somatomedins." These liver hormones are peptides that produce major effects on the growth of bone and muscle. They also influence the metabolism of ingested minerals, including calcium, phosphate, carbohydrates, and lipids (fat). Somatomedin growth factors are indirectly stimulated to divide by the pituitary hormone somatotropin (also referred to as "growth hormone" by endocrinologists).

The peptide growth factors act by binding to functional receptors that transduct their signals and the peptides themselves may be viewed as bifunctional molecules.

The following are two main responses or actions that peptide growth factors accomplish:

(a) They possess an afferent function in that there is the conveying of information to cellular receptors, providing them with information from outside the organism's cell, tissue, or organ.

(b) They have an efferent function in that there is the inception of a latent biochemical activity of the receptor.

107

The Peptide Growth Factors within Liver Cells

A certain piece of geographic knowledge in nature's lore (presented in the paragraph immediately below) perhaps best illustrates how peptide growth factors must be considered cell-to-cell signals, rather than as the equivalents of metallic parts of a machine. They offer up physiological symbols of communication within the organ systems of nearly all animal organisms. Peptides possess the unique action of serving as a significant means to convey information from one cell to another or from one organ to another, including the brain and central nervous system; their action in this regard is contextual.

Natural lore shows us the way peptide growth factors act to convey information inside their animal host. I ask you to visualize the reversal of host animal peptide growth factors communication in the following context:

It's a fact that in two closely located islands off the coast of South Africa, a rock lobster and a large snail have reversed their predator-prey relationships. On island "Gamma," the lobster preys on the snail: finds it, attacks it, and eats its soft parts with gusto. Fifty nautical miles to the east on island "Omega," a reversal of the roles between prey and predator takes place. The same species of snail that had been eaten, now preys on the same species of lobster by approaching it, extending a probing foot, burying that foot into the lobster's body, and sucking out its gizzards. (32)

What produces the reversal in predator-prey relationships? It's the host animals' peptide growth factors. Within each of the animal organisms, their growth factors alter attitude so as to become contextual; they signal differing elements of an intercellular language. To be contextual means that the whole situation, background, or environment becomes relevant to this particular animalistic prey-predator event, as determined by molecular makeup of the participants' peptide growth factors.

Interleukin-6 (IL-6), one of the known peptide growth factors, regulates the protein synthesis in a human being's liver cells (hepatocytes). Also transforming growth factor-beta (TGF-beta), another set of peptide growth factors produced by normal human fibroblasts, additionally regulates the synthesis and secretion of human immunoglobulins by B-lymphocytes. (33-36) Since immune cells also synthesize both TGF-beta and IL-6, these molecules provide a means of communication between the immune system and its immediate neighbors. The liver is part of almost every detoxification process; therefore, the hepatocytes are often significantly involved with the metabolism of neighboring cells.

Inasmuch as the liver's natural function makes it a part of all aspects of physiological repair in the presence of body pathology, the peptide growth factors of the liver cells must be critical determinants of every aspect of tissue trauma or illness response. As such, liver cell peptide growth factors have important and necessary therapeutic applications. The peptide growth factors, whose functions and applications are described below by Stewart Lanson, M.D., of Scottsdale, Arizona and Howard Benedict, D.C., of New York City, bring major impacts to the practice of clinical medicine and nutritional science. These peptide growth factors are involved in the repair of both soft and hard body tissues, immunosuppression, enhancement of immune cellular function, improvement of bone marrow function in numerous disease states, treatment of many proliferative diseases including the remission of cancer, the marked lowering of serum cholesterol, (37) and for the

elimination of all hepatitis viral diseases, but most
especially for hepatitis B and C. (38)

Stuart Lanson, M.D., Treats Hepatitis C
with Liver Peptides

Scottsdale, Arizona clinical ecologist Stuart Lanson,
M.D. is an allergist holding board certification in
environmental medicine. He is the medical director of the
Scottsdale Ear, Nose, Throat, Allergy, and Environmental
Health Center. Regarding treatment with liver peptides, he
says:

> I use the liquid liver peptides for those of
> my patients who are environmentally ill with
> xenobiotics, allopathic hydrocarbons, pesti-
> cides, PCBs, and solvents. All of these toxins
> are stored in body fat, but they can be
> measured in the blood in parts per billion.
>
> For those patients who have problems with
> detoxification, I employ the frozen, liquid
> liver extract as a standard treatment. Also I
> use this extract for those people suffering
> from the various hepatitis illnesses, most
> particularly for viral hepatitis C.
>
> For example, a woman in her early forties
> coming to me from a nearby Arizona city had
> a clear diagnosis of hepatitis C. All of her
> liver enzymes were severely elevated and her
> symptoms included an enlarged, tender liver,
> lethargy, poor appetite, nausea, vomiting,
> fever, joint pains, and jaundice. I put her on
> multiple nutritional supplements, an elevated
> dosage of olive leaf extract, and NatCell™

Liver. I did this in order to have these substances work together against the virus and to strengthen her liver. Also I treated some of her allergies with immunotherapy and preservative-free antigens.

This woman has now dramatically improved. Her liver enzymes have returned to normal levels and her various symptoms have left. She reports having the same normal amount of energy as she had before she contracted hepatitis C. My patient has now returned to work; she has expressed her happiness to me; and she is basically quite well.

I do need to put in the limiting information that most of these hepatitis C patients do not show improvements in their viral counts. The counts continue to remain elevated, even though my patients exhibit wellness and state that they feel better. The viral numbers do not seem to lower significantly," and blood tests indicate that their viruses have not disappeared.

Still, I do treat many hepatitis C patients who respond just fine to the strengthening of their liver organs by their sublingually ingesting the live cell liver treatment. This treatment overcomes their severe fatigue, impaired liver function, and elevated liver enzymes. They see noticeable symptomatic improvement! Invariably the patients' fatigue goes away, and they are able to work once again. Of course, I add other modalities besides the bovine liver growth factors, but

111

these peptides are definitely helpful in repairing damaged liver organs. My finding is that the tiny live proteins repair a damaged liver.

Among the hundreds of clinical journal research reports that can be acquired from an Internet search of Medline, the following are only a few about the great physiological and metabolic advantages made available by liver growth factors. Research on liver growth factors has been conducted both on animals and cultures in laboratories, as well as on sick patients receiving treatment in clinics and medical offices.

From the Department of Internal Medicine at Keio University in Tokyo, Japan, researchers report that a combined preparation of liver growth factors and flavin adenine dinucleotide (FAD) has been widely used for patients with chronic liver disease. In particular, those Japanese suffering with hepatitis C viral infections (HCV) benefited from intravenous injections of this preparation. It seems to be a potent agent for the enhancement of the anti-viral efficacy of interferon (IFN) in patients with chronic hepatitis C (CH-C). (39)

Extracts from the weaning pig liver, although not bovine, also have acted synergistically with hepatocyte growth factors to stimulate improved function of the liver cells. The researchers did report that in the absence of added porcine growth factors, the extracts had no activity.

From the Third Department of Internal Medicine, National Defense Medical College in Saitama, Japan we learn about the peptide growth factor known as Transforming Growth Factors-alpha (TGF-alpha). These particular growth factors cause biological activity when they come in contact with an extract of human exocrine

112

pancreatic cancer associated with humoral hypercalcemia of malignancy. (40)

Two mitogenic pepticles in bovine liver extracts show mitogenesis and other metabolic activity when they come in contact (in the laboratory) with basic fibroblast growth factor (FGF). (41)

Originally described as a hepatocyte peptide specific mitogen, hepatocyte growth factor (HGF) is a potent stimulator of DNA synthesis in a wide variety of cell types. It has the unique ability to transmit information that determines the spatial organization of epithelial cells in tissues as well as induce cell migration and invasion of extracellular matrix in a variety of epithelial cells. HGF is involved in physiological processes such as embryogenesis and development and in pathophysiological processes such as regeneration and carcinogenesis. (42)

Investigations conducted at the University of Alabama in Birmingham, U.S.A. indicate that HGF is an important mediator of interactions for carrying on human mitogenesis, motogenesis, and morphogenesis. (43)

As a mesenchymal-derived morphogen, HGF supports epithelial branching duct formation in the developing lung. It prevents the onset or progress of hepatic fibrosis/cirrhosis and accompanying severe liver failure. HGF may be used successfully as treatment for vascular disease, gastric ulcers, diabetes mellitus, and neuronal disease. (44)

From the Department of Pathology at the University of Pittsburgh, we learn that HGF, epidermal growth factor (EGF), TGF-alpha, IL-6, tumor necrosis factor-alpha (TNF-alpha), insulin, and norepinephrine each play important roles in the sequential changes of gene expression, growth factor production, and morphologic structure. (45)

The Potential Healing Benefits of
Live Cell Liver Peptides

Located under the diaphragm and occupying most of the right hypochondrium and part of the epigastrium of the abdomen, the liver provides vital functions for the body by means of its growth factors.

In preparing for our interview about his use of frozen, liquid, bovine liver peptide growth factors, Dr. Howard Benedict, a nutrition-oriented chiropractor practicing in New York City, discussed with me the potential healing benefits of these frozen liver peptides. In summary, Dr. Benedict offers the following information about the liver's numerous growth factors:

- The growth factors of the liver have vascular functions, in that they cause the liver to store blood, regulate blood clotting, cleanse blood, discharge waste products into the bile, and aid the immune system by filtering the blood to remove bacteria and adding certain immune factors.

- They have secretory functions, in that they aid digestion by synthesizing and secreting bile and keeping hormones in balance.

- They have metabolic functions in that they help to manufacture new proteins, produce quick energy, regulate fat storage, control the production and excretion of cholesterol, store certain vitamins, minerals, and sugars, metabolize alcohol, carbohydrates, proteins, and fat, and proceed with detoxifying, neutralizing, and destroying xenobotic substances such as drugs, pesticides, chemicals, and pollutants.

• They are therapeutic when administered for fatty liver, hepatitis, fibrosis, cirrhosis, and damage to the liver as the result of exposure to internal and environmental toxins.

Dr. Benedict says:

Patients who consulting receive a functional liver assessment or test, and I check their phase one and phase two metabolic liver detoxification processes.

A patient's liver is challenged with caffeine or aspirin to determine its function; and if there is an elevation of enzymes, tissues within the liver designed for detoxification are tested for breakdown. Liver enzyme elevation indicates such tissue breakdown. That being the case, I intervene on behalf of the patient <u>to enhance his or her health and well-being on a functional level, way before there is the onset of disease.</u>

For those people with advanced liver pathology, the usual orthomolecular nutritional treatment protocols such as the taking of vitamin C, alpha lipoic acid, milk thistle, curcuminoids, dandelion, green tea, and others are not enough. The more aggressive and effective treatment required is the NatCell™ Liver. Such therapy helps the patient's liver regenerate. In many situations, especially in chronic illnesses, giving someone a chance by feeding his or her ailing organ the live liver peptide growth factors, taken from a bovine source, does the job.

How to Use the Frozen, Liquid Bovine Peptide Growth Factors

Howard Benedict, D.C., conforms to the manufacturer's suggested instructions for patient and health professional's use of the frozen, liquid extract. The manufacturer's product package insert tells us that the liquid extract is marketed as a food supplement only for oral use and should always be kept frozen. The insert also states:

• Peptides should be taken on an empty stomach in the morning or in the evening, either half an hour before or two hours after a meal.

• They come in a seven-cubic centimeter vial of frozen liquid that should be thawed by holding the vial in the hand.

• Shake the contents of the vial well before unscrewing the vial cap.

• Pour half of the vial's 7 cc-content (3.5 cc) under the tongue. Hold the liquid sublingually for five minutes, and then swallow it.

• Repeat this same action with the second half of liquid.

- Keep the vial closed between each step.

- According to Dr. Benedict, who adheres to the manufacturer's recommendations, use should be as a nutritional supplement at the rate of one or two vials per week.

- This frozen, liquid, bovine liver peptide live cell extract may not be suitable for pregnant or nursing women and children under twelve years of age.

During my treatment I took:

Two 500 mg. liver organic capsules two times per day.
I suggest Natcell liver, two vials per week (optional).

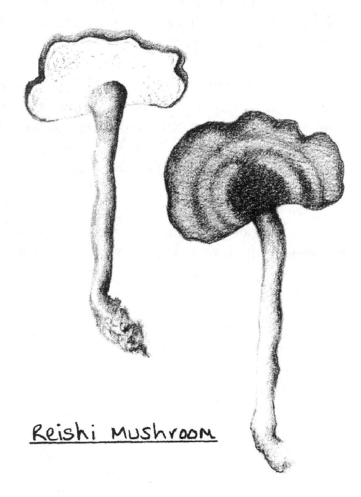

Reishi Mushroom

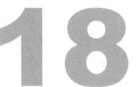

REISHI MUSHROOMS

Reishi mushrooms have been used for thousands of years to promote good health in the Far East. David Law writes:

> The Reishi mushroom can increase the production of interleukin1 and 2, resulting in inhibition of tumor growth. Studies show that Reishi can have a number of other positive effects on the body such as analgesic, anti-inflammatory, antioxidant, anti-viral (through its interferon production), lowers blood pressure. It also acts as a cardiotonic by lowering serum and increasing the production of interleukin 1 and 2, which results in

inhibition of tumor cholesterol, expectorant, anti-tissue, liver protecting and detoxifying, protection against ionizing radiation, antibacterial, and anti-HIV activity. (46)

We live in artificial environments where air is filtered and food is processed. If we can keep our immune system functioning efficiently and strengthen our daily programs with natural immunity building supplements such as Reishi mushrooms, we can minimize the frequency and severity of illness and recover more quickly.

To further mystify your brain into believing that the FDA has not yet graduated from kindergarten: the Chinese Chow Dynasty used Reishi mushrooms. This means that people knew about the healing properties of Reishi mushrooms over three thousand years ago.

The compounds found in Reishi mushrooms have been classified as Host Defense Potentiators (HDP). These enhance the abilities of our immune system to protect itself. These disease-inhibiting compounds include Hemicellulose (AHCC), polysaccharides, polysaccharide-peptides, nucleosides, triterpeniods, complex starches, and other metabolites. In combination they strengthen the immune system, aid in neuron transmission, metabolism, hormonal balance, and the transport of nutrients and oxygen.

I strongly advocate the consumption of natural, unadulterated, non-processed, authentic Reishi mushrooms. Purchase them in bulk, along with a seriously sharp knife for these little guys are very tough. In order to cut one into little pieces, you first must work yourself into a murderous frenzy. Make believe you're an ex-football player and commence to slay the little fungi.

During my treatment I drank:

Two cups of Reishi per day. You may also take Reishi capsules, one 500 mg. three times per day.

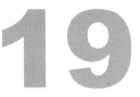

ALPHA-LIPOIC ACID (ALA): A POWERFUL ANTIOXIDANT

Alpha-lipoic acid is an antioxidant used in Europe to restore liver health. It confers protective benefits against oxidative processes involved in degenerative diseases. It is more potent than vitamins C, E, and Co-Q10, and according to Dr. Ester Packer, professor of molecular biology at UC Berkley, alpha-lipoic acid may be the most important antioxidant ever discovered:

> Vitamins C, E and glutathione work together to deactivate and prevent free radicals from causing uncontrolled damage in the body. But at this stage we run into a limiting factor regarding availability of

glutathione, which is an important free-radical deactivator offering protection against cataract formation, as well as immune enhancement, liver protection, cancer protection, and heavy-metal detoxification.

When taken orally like Vitamins C and E, glutathione is broken down in the stomach before it reaches the bloodstream. What does end up being absorbed can raise serum levels, but the effect inside of the cells is minimal.

Alpha-lipoic acid is the missing link. Not only is ALA a powerful antioxidant in its own right, but it also regenerates glutathione, giving cells a double dose of antioxidant protection. In addition, it is easily absorbed when taken orally, and once inside cells it is quickly converted to its most potent form, dihydrolipoic acid, which is an even more potent free-radical neutralizer than ALA. Because both alpha-lipoic acid and dihydrolipoic acid are antioxidants, their combined actions give them greater antioxidant potency than any other natural antioxidant now known.

Scientists have also found that lipoic acid can inhibit replication of HIV-1 and other viruses through its ability to bind directly to DNA. (47)

Dr. Packer and Chandan K. Sen, a researcher from Finland, have described how alpha-lipoic acid regulates aspects of the immune system, and in particular, immune cells called T-lymphocytes. These two researchers, along with other scientists, have reported how alpha-lipoic acid may help people with HIV:

> ALA inhibits growth of HIV more effectively than NAC (N-Acetyl Cysteine) ....alpha-lipoic acid completely inhibited activation of a gene in the AIDS virus that allows it to reproduce.

Early in 1995, shortly after my diagnosis of hepatitis C, I was consulting my brother Dwain about my will. Dwain exists in Oregon in a somewhat unusual way. Apparently he has a radio, for it was Dwain who told me he was listening to a doctor on a talk radio program out of Seattle, who was treating hepatitis C with 50,000 mg. injections of Vitamin C twice daily in combination with alpha-lipoic acid. ALA is a co-factor in the multi-enzyme complex that catalyzes the last stage of the process called glycolysis.

Please keep in mind, I'm not a doctor. I am a patient, who was very disappointed after spending a fortune trying to get information from doctors, and who then set out on my own to save my life. I'm sure many readers won't realize what a horrendous quest this was or how devastated I was by what I discovered about our institutions.

I may write things you find offensive, while others may find them quite hilarious. I don't mean to transmit any insults; this is just the way I see it. Being at the "DOOR OF DEATH" is very different than merely contemplating it.

Truth is stranger than fiction. This book is about truth. It's about me. I'm well; I tested negative for hepatitis C on April 10, 1997. My last test was on October 5, 2001. The results were as follows: PCR HCV RNA QUANTA-TATIVE NON-DETECTED. ALT 13; AST 17.

The remedy I put before you worked for me, and it has proven to be successful on several hundred others. Healers have used many parts of this remedy all over the world since ancient times. A very small segment of health care professionals – including naturopaths, acupuncturists, chiropractors, and other kinds of holistic healers – have also learned things beyond what the FDA allows.

Alpha-lipoic acid occurs naturally in potatoes, sweet potatoes, carrots, yams, and red meat. I take additional alpha-lipoic acid every day, and know it has been vital in my battle and success with hepatitis C.

During my treatment I took:

Two 100 mg. lipoic acid capsules two times per day. Today, I suggest taking one 200 mg. lipoic acid capsule three times per day.

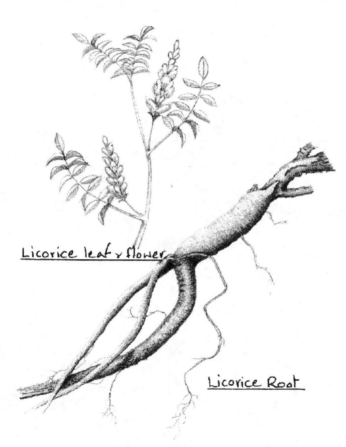

Licorice leaf & flower

Licorice Root

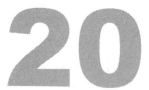

LICORICE ROOT:
A BIOLOGICALLY ACTIVE HERB

Licorice was brought to my attention by Candy, who works at Pacific Coast Greens, a great health food store in Malibu. I've done some research on it, using myself as a guinea pig. I found licorice to be a wonderful herb, for it does away with all sorts of uncomfortable nuisances, including high temperature, ulcers, and arthritis.

Dan Mowrey states:

> Licorice root is one of the most biologically active herbs in the world. Licorice root is an effective treatment for stomach ailments, because it exerts a soothing action on the mucosal surfaces of the GI tract, and it is frequently used to help these tissues heal.

129

The licorice root derivatives, glycryuhetinic acid (GLA), deglycrihyinated licorice (DGL), and carbenoxolene sodium (CS) have all been proven to be among the best anti-ulcer medications available. Whole licorice and its derivatives appear to have the ability to inhibit gastric acid secretion with the advantage of being devoid of other adverse anti-cholinergic properties.

Licorice root helps prevent and heal skin problems. The conditions that increase the occurrence of acne-like symptoms during certain stages of the menstrual cycle may be affected by the consumption of licorice root.

The anti-inflammatory properties of the root have been considered responsible for its effectiveness in the treatment of numerous skin disorders, including eczema, dermatitis, impetigo, and traumatized skin.

It should be mentioned that the antipyrelic (fever reducing) effects of GLA have been shown to be equal to those of the widely used sodium salicylate. (48)

Fever reduction is important to hepatitis C patients. My experience for several years was that I was always at about 99.8 degrees. My fever would rise after eating. It was extremely uncomfortable to live day after day, year after year, just a little bit hot.

Every time a doctor would record my slightly elevated temperature, I would ask why it was high. The usual answer was, "you probably just have a bug." Taking licorice really helped this problem.

Licorice root is used to remove buildup of toxic metabolic substances in the body, because it increases the liver's ability to filter out these wastes.

In the treatment of liver diseases (e.g. hepatitis and cirrhosis), GLA has proven extremely promising. In Chinese medicine, licorice is often used as a remedy for jaundice and is considered a great liver detoxifier. According to Dan Mowry:

> Experimental work has validated the usefulness of licorice in the treatment of hepatitis, cirrhosis, and related liver disorders. Licorice is a good tonic for the adrenal glands and Addison's disease.

This is very important for the hepatitis C patient because you need to support your adrenal gland in many ways in order to conquer the virus.

Mowrey continues:

> Licorice appears to both mimic and potentiate the action of the adrenal-caiticosteroids, though it also differs in action from these chemicals in several important ways.
>
> Licorice components have been found to exert a positive effect on the course of several adrenal insufficiencies, even in Addison's disease, which is characterized by near total adrenal exhaustion.

In later stages, the hepatitis C patient may develop severe joint pain, which I did. This pain was compounded one hundred fold by interferon. Mowrey writes:

> The anti-arthritic properties of GLA and the aqueous extracts of licorice have also been shown. Comparisons of licorice root to hydrocortisone are frequently made in the medical literature in England, China, and countries other than the USA.
>
> In relation to the immune system, (which hepatitis C patients must become obsessed with boosting), licorice root and its derivatives have recently shown extremely promising results as interferon inducers, which is especially good news for the treatment of hepatitis C. (When was the last time your hepatitis C doctor told you that)?
>
> At concentrations well tolerated by uninfected cells, glycyrhezic acid inhibits both growth and cytopathic effect of vaccinia, as well as herpes simplex, Newcastle disease, and vesicular stomatits viruses while being ineffective on polio virus.

It is suggested that glycyrhezic acid interacts with virus structures (conservable proteins) producing different effects according to the viral stage affected: inactivation of free virus particles extracellularly; prevention of intercellular uncoating of infecting particles; impairment of the assembling ability of virus structural components. Dr. Mowry further states:

As a general cautionary measure, persons with a history of hypertension, renal failure, or who are currently using cardiac glycosides may wish to avoid the use of licorice root altogether.

During my treatment I took:

One 500 mg. licorice capsule two times per day, five days a week. I also drank two cups of licorice tea five days a week.

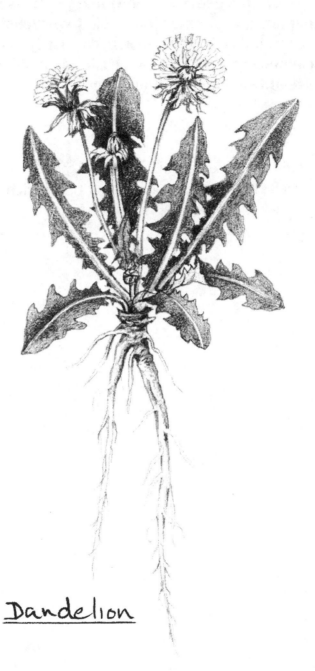

Dandelion

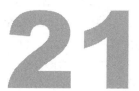

DANDELION ROOT:
A NATURAL LIVER TONIC

The first mention of the dandelion as a medicinal plant was in writings by Arabian physicians of the Tenth and Eleventh Centuries. Today dandelions are cultivated primarily in India as a remedy for liver disease.

The dandelion is a perennial plant found almost everywhere, to the dismay of many. Its properties and uses include: aperient, cholague, diuretic, and tonic.

In his book *The Herb* Book, John Lust writes:

> The dandelion has two particularly important uses; to promote the formation of bile and to remove excess water from the body in edema conditions resulting from liver

135

problems. By acting to remove poisons from the body, it acts as a tonic and stimulant. The fresh juice is most effective, but dandelion is also prepared as a tea. An infusion of the fresh root is said to be good for gallstones, jaundice, and other liver problems. (49)

While I was undergoing radiation therapy for cancer, my liver count alarmed the doctor. He insisted I must be a drug addict and severe alcoholic. I begged to differ with him. On several occasions he argued with me, attempting to get me to admit something that wasn't true.

My mother, a health food fanatic of the 1950's, always told me dandelions were good for my liver. When I remembered what my mother told me about dandelions, I began drinking two quarts of dandelion tea a day. I told the Oncologist, and he insisted that there was nothing I could take that would lower my liver count. That I should just stop drinking and using drugs.

After one month of drinking two quarts of dandelion tea a day, my ALT count dropped fifty points. Since then, I've been taking dandelion root everyday.

During my treatment I took:

One 500 mg. organic dandelion root capsule three times per day. I also made dandelion root tea and drank one quart every evening.

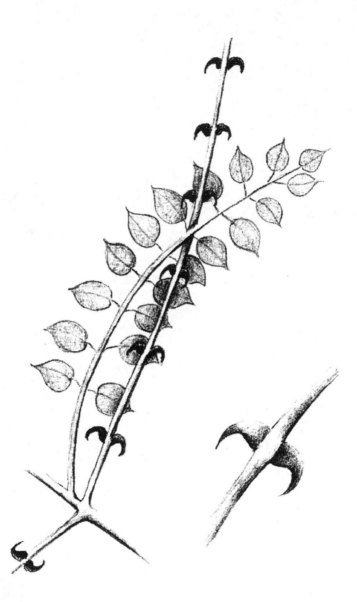

Cat's Claw

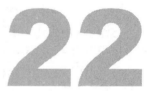

CAT'S CLAW
(UNCARIA TAMENTOSA):
A POTENT CELLULAR
RECONSTITUTOR

Cat's claw is an herb that grows in the rain forest of the Peruvian Amazon. Native Peruvian Indians have used it for centuries, dating back to the ancient Incas. The inner bark contains unique active constituents to help support the body's natural defenses.

Cat's claw is currently the subject of extensive scientific research and is used worldwide as a nutritional supplement.

I discovered Cat's claw on the internet while desperately seeking a cure for hepatocellular carcinoma. When he informed me of my hepatitis C infection, the

139

blood donor bank technician offered the possibility that I might die from this disease. He suggested that my final demise would be from this form of cancer, because there was no possible way to alter the death path of hepatitis C. Mickey Mantle, Alan Ginsburg, and many other famous people have died from hepatocellular carcinoma, as a complication of hepatitis C.

Unknown to most Americans, Cat's claw is labeled as a cancer cure and sold over the counter in most South American countries. It has terrific anti-viral qualities as well and should not be overlooked in your quest for life.

Six oxindole alkaloids have been isolated from the inner bark. These oxindole alkaloids have been proven to provide a general boost to the immune system and have a profound effect on the ability of white blood cells to engulf and digest harmful microorganisms and foreign matter. Other alkaloids and phytochemicals present in Cat's claw have been shown to provide natural support against many viruses.

Besides containing oxindole alkaloids, Peruvian and Italian researchers have discovered a wealth of other beneficial phytochemicals inherent in the herb, including proanthacyanidens, polyphenols, triterpines and plant sterols beta-stitosterol, stigmasterol and campesterol. The presence of these additional compounds might further explain the anti-oxidant, anti-microbial, anti-tumor and anti-inflammatory properties attributed to this herb. It is a powerful cellular reconstitutor.

In the words of Dr. Brent Davis:

> Uncaria Tomentosa (Cat's claw) is a world-class herb which has the power to arrest and reverse deep-seated pathology, allowing a

more rapid return to health in the context of consistent A. K. therapies. (50)

During my treatment I took:

Two 500 mg. cat's claw capsules two times per day. I also drank two cups of cat's claw tea per day.

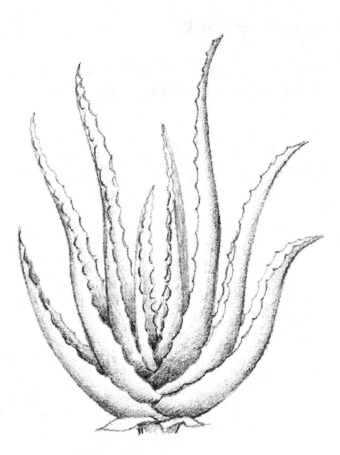

Aloe Vera

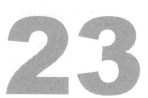

ALOE VERA: HOLISTICALLY PERFECT PLANT

According to Dr. John Finnegan, mucopolysaccharides are made in the human body and perform many key functions in our health, including growth and immune system functioning. Unfortunately, after puberty we cease manufacturing mucopolysaccharides and must obtain them from outside sources. Mucopolysaccharides are found in large amounts in fresh aloe vera and in properly prepared aloe vera juices. Following are a few of the vital functions this substance has been found to perform.

- They become incorporated into the cellular membrane and make the cell more resistant to viruses and pathogenic bacteria.

- They improve overall cellular metabolism and functioning.

- They have anti-inflammatory properties.

- They provide critical lubrication of joints; helping to prevent arthritis and to heal it once it has developed.

- They aid in the absorption of water, minerals, and nutrients in the GI track.

- They improve macrophage (white blood cells) activity making them up to ten times more effective in engulfing foreign matter.

- They enhance the macrophage's effectiveness in modulating the entire immune system.

- They enhance the macrophage's effectiveness to stimulate and direct the production and release of antibodies (increasing the body's own production of interferon, interleukins and more).

- They increase the number of antibody forming T-cells in the spleen and increase the number and activity of killer T-cell and monocyte activity.

- They are responsible for aloe's special penetration properties.

- In conjunction with their cellular detoxification support and immune enhancement, they improve allergic reactions.

- They stimulate bone marrow activity.

- They stimulate the fibroblasts to release collagen and elastin to make new tissue (inside and out).

- The mucopolysaccharides in aloe vera enhance the functioning of the entire immune system, and repair and detoxify the digestive and elimination systems of the body. (51)

Dr. John Finnegan prescribed aloe vera for me, and at the time I had no idea that it was anything more than expensive cactus juice. After taking it for two days, the diarrhea I'd had most of the time since my four blood transfusions was gone. There was a true feeling of reversal from sicker and sicker to a leveling off and a healing taking place. Of course, Dr. John Finnegan prescribed several other things in the first few months, only a few of which I could afford. Aloe vera was one item I purchased by the case from him. He has had great successes in using aloe with his hepatitis clients. Properly prepared aloe vera is a must in the quest against hepatitis C. In chronic hepatitis C cases there is suffering from severe joint pain. Aloe vera helped eliminate this pain for me better than anything else I've tried. The cost can drive you to the poor house, but at least the physical suffering on the way isn't as bad. Wouldn't it be great if you were one of those fortunate enough to have insurance and they would pay for at least a portion of this product? It's better than most things you'll ever buy in a bottle.

145

The FDA allows aloe vera companies to label their products "cold pressed" if they are kept under 400 degrees. However, heating aloe vera over 90 degrees shortens the mucopolysaccharide molecule. Most of the aloe on the shelves in health food stores has been heated. Herbal Aloe Force is one of the companies that guarantee, in writing, that their aloe is never heated!

John Pittman, M.D. writes in *The Immune Enhancing Effects of Aloe*:

Beta-glucomannans are a class of very long chain sugars derived from plants, which have been shown in laboratory and clinical studies to have a wide variety of immune stimulating and protective effects within the body. In studying the different sources of this polymer, it has been discovered that the aloe barbadensis plant contains the greatest concentration of acetylated polymannans, which is also the most active form of mannans. These long-chain complex polysaccharides are often called beta-glucomannans, mucopolysaccharides or Acemannan. These aloe polysaccharides have been shown to have many effects in the body, mostly impacting the gastrointestinal and immune systems, which are intricately related. Before elaborating on their beneficial effects, it is appropriate to discuss the type of pathology often present in individuals experiencing immune system depression.

146

The most striking commonality found in individuals suffering with immune depressive conditions such as Epstein-Barr virus, chronic fatigue syndrome, systemic candidiasis, HIV infection and others, is the high incidence of digestive dysfunction and maldigestion. This has several effects that contribute to stress on the immune system and weakening it.

Maldigestion means that the consumed food is not properly broken down into the elemental building blocks needed for the body to rebuild itself and to generate energy for metabolism. This results in a type of starvation at the cellular level, with all tissue suffering malnourishment and therefore decreased effectiveness of all internal chemical processes.

These processes include breakdown and transport of toxins out of the cell, movement of nutrients into the cell, and energy production for cell functioning. This affects all the cells in the body, including those of the immune system such as white blood cells, (macrophages, and lymphocytes) and red blood cells, which carry oxygen throughout our bodies. Not only do we lack enough fuel, but we're low on oxygen too.

However, it is not this cellular starvation alone that causes the immune depression. Maldigestion also results in pathologic reactions. First, these remnants become irritants and cause inflammation of the mucosal wall of the intestines. Many powerful enzymes and damaging chemicals are released, injuring the intestinal wall causing increased intestinal mucosal permeability. The foreign proteins of the digested food can leak across the mucosa into the lymphatic channels of the intestinal wall and from there, gain access to the circulatory system. Here, these absorbed proteins are recognized as foreign and are attacked by the cells of the immune system. Antibodies bind to the protein and then call in the macrophages and monocytes. T-cells arrive later, releasing enzymes and using oxygen to drive the metabolic breakdown of the foreign protein. The total result is that the immune system is constantly turned on and draining down like a battery. As these allergic reactions to food breakdown products continue, the cells of the immune system wear out faster, run out of fuel and aren't reproduced in sufficient numbers.

In addition to this chronic hyper-immune state, undigested food remnants provide fuel for overgrowth of fermentative fungal organisms such as Candida Albicans as well as several types of parasites. Overgrowth of Candida in the intestines has significant effects throughout the body due to the absorption of toxic by-products of its metabolism. This can result in worsening of food allergies, hypoglycemia, digestive disturbances, excessive mucus, bloating, flatulence, skin rashes, and extreme fatigue. This chronic infection further drains the immune system and complicates the picture.

Further damage is inflicted on all cell membranes from the effects of the generalized inflammation occurring as a result of maldigestion. These metabolic reactions utilize large amounts of oxygen and produce oxidative free radicals as waste by-products. The negatively charged oxygen molecules are desperately trying to balance their electrical charge and immediately begin to chop holes into cell membranes as they grab positive charges. The result here is further damage to the intestinal mucosa and a worsening of the increased permeability.

All these processes work together in a vicious sequence of events leading to progressive weakening of the immune system. It is clear that many mechanisms are at play in orchestrating these processes. Without definitive therapy directed at each component of the immune system pathology, this is a downward spiral to death. Fortunately, a thorough multidimensional treatment protocol addressing each component has been shown to reverse these processes. Aloe vera has been shown to have properties addressing all these issues and appears to play a key role on many different levels in boosting all immune functioning.

At the intestinal level, the aloe polysaccharides have been shown to act as potent anti-inflammatory agents, neutralizing many of the enzymes responsible for damaging the mucosal wall and, in effect, quenching the fire. They do this anti-inflammatory action while at the same time boosting the immune system functioning. This results in decreased leakiness of the intestinal wall and less absorption of allergic stimulating foreign protein as well as enhancing the repair of the tissue. Research has also demonstrated their direct viricidal, bactericidal, and fungicidal properties, which can help control Candida overgrowth so the normal gastrointestinal bacterial flora can be restored. It has also been found that these polysaccharides stimulate intestinal motility, improving the elimination process to move allergenic proteins from the small intestine into the colon. All these processes help to normalize gastrointestinal wall structure and function and therefore stop the viscous cycle of immune system damage.

In addition to restoring gastrointestinal and elimination functioning, large glucomannan polysaccharides also have direct effects on the cells of the immune system.

They have been shown to increase the number of and activate the intensity of macrophages, monocytes, and T-cells as well as increasing the number of antibody forming B-cells in the spleen. Enhancing macrophage activity increases the effectiveness of the entire immune and repair system of the body as it is responsible for so many functions, including immune modulation.

These polysaccharides have been shown in laboratory studies to act as a bridge between foreign proteins (such as virus particles) and the macrophage, facilitating phagocytosis ingestion of the protein by the macrophage. Activating the receptor sites of the macrophages is a key to the overall boosting of cell-mediated immunity, which is deficient in HIV infection and other immune disorders. These aloe polysaccharides also protect the bone marrow from damage by toxic chemicals and drugs.

These various effects, while seemingly wide spread and unrelated, are in fact due to one simple process at the cell membrane level. Acemannan (the name often used for aloe beta-glucomannans, acetylated polymannans and mucopolysaccharides) is a long chain sugar that interjects itself into all cell membranes. This results in an increase in the fluidity and permeability of the membranes allowing toxins to flow out of the cell more easily and nutrients to enter the cell. This results in improved cellular metabolism throughout the body and an overall boost in energy production. The vicious cycle of maldigestion and cellular starvation is finally broken as the Acemannan normalizes absorption of nutrients and increases tolerance for allergenic foods (from detoxification). The immune system is now stronger, under control, and better prepared for any new threat.

As humans living in the late twentieth century, our body's metabolic and detoxification systems are under ever increasing stress from foreign chemicals, nutrient depleted foods, and immune damaging infectious agents.

In order to control and prevent the inevitable progression of the immune system destruction that these stresses cause, therapy must be multifactorial involving all levels of health, diet and lifestyle. These different areas consist of destruction of pathogenic organisms, metabolic detoxification, intestinal cleansing, increasing cellular metabolism, antioxidant agents to combat free radicals, and direct stimulation of immune system cells. Aloe vera's Acemannan, the active ingredient in cold-processed, whole leaf aloe, has been demonstrated in laboratory testing and clinical use to be effective on all levels of this therapeutic program. (52)

Jeri L. Heyman, Ph.D. writes in *The Secret Promise of Aloe Vera:*

I am a developmental psychologist who has focused on psychological and emotional development for most of my life and career. By becoming aware of the latest research on aloe vera, I have become inspired to examine healthy physical development more closely in addition to the biochemical contribution to overall optimal health and balance. I found the aloe vera plant to be the most fascinating and miraculous plant on the planet. I have spent the last five years investigating aloe vera, and it keeps getting more interesting all the time. As you begin to look at the information on aloe, you may find conflicting information. Please be aware that there is still a great deal of misinformation and misunderstandings about aloe vera and aloe vera products. It is very hard to believe that all the scientific research on the properties of fresh aloe vera could possibly be real - but they are.

The research raised many questions for me. How could something be so profoundly and fundamentally effective for so many areas of health and have only good side effects? Why (if this research is real and aloe has been around for so long) haven't we heard more about experiences of these miraculous effects? What I found is that the research on fresh aloe vera is real and the research on the constituents in fresh aloe is real. However, most of the aloe vera products available in the marketplace are not demonstrating the promises documented by the research, even though they have some benefits. Thus, aloe vera's true potential has remained a secret. (53)

The Effectiveness of Aloe Vera – Fundamental and Profound.

The Immune System:

Scientific research has demonstrated so many healthful properties of aloe that one's immediate response has to be, "this can't be real." Aloe vera enhances the body's own health and healing in so many ways that I wouldn't even have dreamed to pray for them all. Certainly I couldn't have imagined that they would be found all in one plant, in a natural form and with only good side effects.

Fresh aloe vera contains over 250 constituents including the full range of all sizes of polysaccharides (complex sugar chains that feed the cells). The largest long-chain polysaccharides have an intricate, multifaceted, multi-functional biological design and are manufactured by the body only until puberty. After puberty we must get these health and growth producing polysaccharides from outside sources. Aloe vera has been found to be the most concentrated plant source of these largest known and most profound health supporting polysaccharides - the beta-glucomannans (also known as mucopolysaccharides, Acemannan, and acetylated polymannose).

Research by a pharmaceutical company, Carrington Laboratories, has documented some of the astounding properties of the various sizes of the aloe vera long-chain sugars. As reported by Dr. Ivan Danhof, they discovered that the smaller-chained polysaccharides have properties that help in balancing blood sugar levels. Although this is still being studied, there is evidence that they improve insulin receptor cells, with importance for both Type I and Type II diabetes (not to mention balancing sugar cravings). The research has also demonstrated some anti-inflammatory properties of these smaller polysaccharides as they mimic the action of steroids. The medium size polysaccharides have been found to be potent antioxidants. The larger chains have demonstrated direct antibacterial properties (staph, strep, E coli, etc.), direct antiviral properties (herpes, influenza, HIV) and the stimulation of the body's own tissue regeneration processes (by fitting receptor sites of fibroblasts stimulating them to produce collagen and other factors needed to make new tissue).

The largest longest-chained polysaccharides, the beta-glucomannans (mucopolysaccharides), have received the most attention and Carrington has patented the beta 1, 4 glucomannan under the name "Acemannan." They documented astounding immune enhancing and tissue production properties of this aloe polysaccharide. They actually showed that when the Acemannan meets the receptor sites of macrophages it stimulates the macrophage into action and can increase its affectivity ten fold. The macrophages are the main immune system cells. They are the white blood cells that engulf foreign matter throughout the body, release growth factor to stimulate tissue generation, modulate the inflammation processes, and more. They command the other immune cells to release their antibodies – how much, when, and where needed.

Carrington's research showed that when the macrophage is stimulated it does increase the production and release of interferon and the interleukins when needed. This fascinates me because here is a natural way that actually helps the body's own mechanisms to increase antibody production as well as increase the effectiveness of getting to where it's needed. **The body was designed with all the mechanisms to heal itself.** Here there is a way to enhance the body's own systems for healing! The macrophages are also responsible for orchestrating and modulating all the other immune cells and the functioning of the entire immune system. They command the immune cell army, signaling where to go, when and how hard to attack and when to cease-fire.

The question of how can one polysaccharide be so great in so many areas is partly answered here because the macrophage does so many profound things and the beta-glucomannan is making it ten times more effective. So, when the literature on aloe vera talks about direct immune enhancement, they are referring to this body of research on polysaccharides by Carrington Laboratories.

Supporting Fundamental Health
By "Re-Naturing" the Cells.

Macrophage stimulation and direct immune system support is just part of the story of how aloe can have such a broad range of health benefits. Aloe vera is known to be the most penetrating and absorbing of substances. It permeates cells and tissues like no other substance on earth. Research has shown that fresh aloe will absorb through to all seven layers of skin. Understanding this action has profound implications understanding the effects of aloe for cellular health. The aloe, led by the large polysaccharide, is of a unique size and shape as to be able to penetrate cell walls dramatically. Sometimes the polysaccharides can become part of the cell membrane fortifying the cell wall. Sometimes the aloe moves into a cell, bringing with it all its nutrients and co-factors. It also cleanses the cells by taking toxins out. The aloe feeds, nourishes, fortifies, and cleanses the cell, improving cellular metabolism and the cell's optimal functioning. I call this "Re-Naturing" the cell because it can feed the cell in such a way as to make it function as it was originally designed by nature. The health benefits of this one property of fresh aloe are mind-boggling. Here is a plant that can improve the health of the cells throughout the body. When the cells are healthy and functioning as they should, all the tissues, glands, organs, and systems of the body are also getting "Re-Natured."

A Myriad of Nutrients and Co-Factors supporting overall Healthy Functioning.

Dr. Robert Davis has done a great deal of research on fresh aloe vera, the properties of its many nutrients, and how the aloe polysaccharides work. Research has found that in addition to the full range of sizes of polysaccharides, fresh aloe contains over 250 other constituents including: vitamins (the only plant source of vitamin B12); minerals, amino acids, essential fatty acids, a natural form of salicylic acid and plant sterols (with antiseptic, anti-inflammatory and analgesic properties), two enzymes that the body needs of which aloe is the only plant source, glycoproteins, and more. These constituents have properties of their own as well as serve as co-factors and support for many of the body's biochemical processes. Dr. Davis' research, as explained below, shows that all the nutrients in aloe vera are crucial to the aloe polysaccharides' effectiveness and biological availability throughout the body.

Isolated Nutrients Extracted by Science Versus The Original Designs Created by Nature.

Carrington Laboratories isolated and patented Acemannan. They continued their research with orally ingested capsules of Acemannan, which was isolated from freeze-dried aloe. The clinical results must not have given them the results they expected, because they switched to the study of injectible Acemannan for which they have FDA approval for study with animals and humans. What does this tell us? I can't imagine that a pharmaceutical

157

company would rather patent an injectible over a capsule. It certainly made me wonder that maybe the research findings only are experienced if the polysaccharides are injected right into where they are needed.

Is this why we haven't heard of these miraculous immune enhancing effects? Is it because the digestive system destroys the polysaccharides? Is it because the polysaccharides can't get through to the lymph system?

It is Dr. Davis' explanation of his "Conductor/Orchestra Theory" that helped me to understand aloe's "Secret Promise." Dr. Davis describes how the entire aloe molecule, with the polysaccharides laced in perfect balance with the other myriad of constituents within a base of water, is what is necessary for the aloe polysaccharides to be available throughout the body and to effectively demonstrate the research on the polysaccharides. The polysaccharide acts as the conductor of the orchestra of all other nutrients. It is the entire "orchestra" that is responsible for the benefits of aloe's "being heard" throughout the body.

As I understand it, the aloe molecule is balanced with the polysaccharide on one end and the other constituents as the "orchestra" on the other end, making it slightly charged on each end. In this form the aloe moves through tissue and throughout the body with the biological design that has a biological wisdom and intercellular communication properties. The aloe works its way to special receptor sites in the digestive tract that ingests the aloe led by the largest polysaccharides and brings it in its whole form into the lymph system where it is then available to move throughout the body and know exactly where to go. Our immune cells send out chemotaxic signals when they are in need of assistance that other immune cells as well as the whole aloe are drawn to.

Thus, it is in its whole form that the aloe polysaccharides are most biologically active and biologically available to the cells of the body. The isolated polysaccharide lacks the biological wisdom and ability to move throughout the body to the cells in need. Thus, the properties of polysaccharides that are not in their original design within the aloe will only work when they happen to hit on particular cells.

It is of critical importance that the aloe not only contain the full range of sizes of polysaccharides but that they also need to be in their originally designed form and balance. Thus, the full promise of aloe vera with all the properties that the research has documented will only be fully demonstrated if the aloe vera is intact.

Why Aloe Vera's True Promise has Been Hidden.

So, again, I ask myself - if this research is real then why aren't we hearing more about these miraculous effects of drinking aloe vera? And why are the aloe vera gels on the market just okay and not the miraculous tissue regenerating gel that the research suggests?

Processing, Processing, Processing! It dawned on me when I used two different aloe juice products that were labeled the exact same way – whole leaf, cold processed, aloin removed – but they tasted different, and they were not equally effective. As my aloe investigation and search for a good aloe product continued, I learned that it is important to read labels very carefully – what they say and do not say are both important.

It makes sense that if the fresh, whole aloe works then we need an aloe that is as close to fresh as possible.

Processed Aloe Vera Versus
Its Original Biological Design.

Although the research is real, the effectiveness of any given aloe product will depend on what "is in" and what "is not in" a given product. Demonstration of the scientific research's promises will depend on having the full range of sizes of polysaccharides in the form they need to be to work best in the body. Thus, any processing of the aloe (to stabilize and purify it) needs to capture and protect all the constituents as well as maintain their original design and balance. Beware of an aloe product that does not guarantee – in writing – that no heat is ever applied from field to bottle. Beware of concentrated or dried aloes. The processing can damage constituents as well as lose their original proportions and design. Aloin is a bitter substance found in Aloe that has unwanted, irritating, laxative properties and is responsible for the contraindications for daily use. Be sure your aloe juice has the aloin removed to less than 1 ppm (laxation occurs at around 2 ppm).

Heat and Biological Activity.

Heat can be the most damaging to the important aloe nutrients. Heat can break down the links between the sugars. When this happens, the long chain sugars no longer have the same size and shape of the polysaccharides that fit the receptor sites of key immune cells and tissue producing cells, nor do they have the other properties that the research has documented.

Heat also breaks down the structure of the enzymes and can also damage amino acids and all the other nutrients. Cells are designed with a biological structure that breaks down with heat above body temperature. As I understand it, the body produces fever, when all else is failing, that helps to kill cells, but unlike other aspects of the immune system, heat does not discriminate between our own cells and foreign cells. Thus, it seems logical that temperatures of 100F- 110F are designed to kill the biological activity (life) of cells in our own bodies. I used to think a fever was a side effect of the body not having enough energy to effectively fight off an illness. But that doesn't make sense to me anymore. If the body has no energy for maintaining the homeostasis (balance) of temperature, it is more likely that the body's temperature would drop. When the immune system is being overtaxed and failing it fires up and uses heat to help to break down and destroy the biological structure for life and growth.

This focus on fever highlights the importance of biological temperatures. When aloe vera (or any food) is heated, intricate biological structures are destroyed along with their biological benefits. Additionally, when aloe vera is heated, not only are the important polysaccharides, enzymes and other factors destroyed, but the balance of the entire aloe molecule is destroyed, and thus its biological availability and effectiveness throughout the body.

Our Bodies are Perfectly Designed.

Our body is designed in perfect balance to take in, absorb and eliminate nutrients and process and eliminate foreign and toxic matter, fight off ills, repair tissue and grow. If given the proper tools, the body is designed to be healthy and strong. The best thing we could do for our bodies is to feed it the nutrients it needs, limit the toxins we take in, not overtax any one system, and protect the balance of all the systems. So look at what we are doing: we do not eat enough raw organic foods that contain the nutrients we need in the form we need them; we eat mostly cooked foods which changes the nutrients into forms that not only do not give the body what it needs, but they burden the body. By age five, the toxins in our environment have overtaxed all the systems of our bodies, and we take medicines that put the digestive system out of balance and do nothing to restore balance and healthy functioning, thus starting a domino effect of problems that eventually overtax the entire immune system's functioning.

All illness can be traced to the body's own systems not working well. Medicine is designed to be crisis intervention (and I am grateful for this) not nutritional health support. We need to learn ways to work with our bodies to support the perfectly designed systems we are. When we treat only the symptoms of illness, we can be interfering with our natural "wellness" processes. Often we are counteracting the body's own wisdom and mechanisms for health. Is diarrhea a sign of illness? Yes and no. Yes, it is a sign that the body is overloaded with waste that needs to be flushed. But no, it is a sign of wellness in that it is flushing the waste from successful immune warfare. Diarrhea is not an illness, per se. It is a result of the body's fighting an illness caused by harmful microorganisms. What an ingenious wellness system: when the fluids from the fight (mucous) build up, the body takes water and mucous from the system and flushes the toxins out.

Enough on that system, let's move on. Think about the mucous produced with allergies and viruses. It is a waste product that needs to be eliminated. We need to help the body get rid of the mucous, not stop it from coming out. When we stop the mucous elimination process, what happens to the toxic waste? We don't need things to dry up the mucous, but we could use a "flush button" that would get rid of it in 5 minutes! I wish all the resources available to medical science were actually focused on wellness!

Our environment and the foods we eat overtax our body's ability to eliminate toxins. Traditional approaches to health care and medicine not only can destroy the digestive system, but also overtax the elimination system, especially the liver. When we stop the symptoms of an illness, we are clogging up the body's immune and elimination systems' natural processes. We can be stopping the body's natural wellness process trying to rid the body of toxic waste. When we do this, we end up overloading the other systems of elimination, especially the kidneys and liver even more.

Aloe Vera – The Herbal Answer to Today's Health Crisis.

Aloe vera is the best herbal answer I can imagine to support the health and healing mechanisms of the body because it doesn't heal, rather, it FEEDS THE BODY'S OWN SYSTEMS in order for them to function optimally and be healthy. It does this, in part, by going into the cells and "Re-Naturing" them to function optimally, as they were originally designed. Thus, aloe is a fundamental tool that gives life to the cells, tissues, glands, organs, and other systems of the body in order to support optimal health, balance, and functioning. In addition, aloe vera has been shown to have many specific properties that profoundly enhance the functioning of body's own immune and repair systems for health and healing to be up to ten times more effective, thus healing can be ten times faster. Aloe vera is a remarkable plant. I urge everyone to examine this for him or her self. To understand that nutrients designed by nature were designed to feed our body perfectly is to understand the importance of feeding the body the fuel it needs to function optimally, as it was originally designed.

The promise in the aloe vera plant has opened my eyes to the need to look at nature's original design for life - to feed life, development and health. It is as though GOD put the aloe vera plant here not only as a gift for health, but also as a metaphor for the miracles that are possible if we trust the design of the divine.

It is fortunate that the aloe vera recommended to me by Dr. Finnegan happened to be a unique aloe product that was enhanced with fantastic immune herbs and processed in a special way. You just can't get any aloe product. Processing will determine what is "in" and "what's not in" the aloe and will determine the results. Once again it is difficult to know the truth about products. So make sure your aloe company guarantees – in writing – that heat is never applied from field to bottle, that it never experiences temperatures above 90F at any time during processing, that it has never been concentrated or diluted, that the whole leaf is being used (more potent), and that the aloin (which can irritate the bowel) is completely removed to 1 ppm or less without any damaging processing. Remember, if it's not written on the bottle, you can't assume anything.

During my treatment I drank:

Four oz. of properly prepared aloe vera two to four times per day, usually more. By properly prepared I mean raw (unheated), organic, whole leaf and never concentrated or diluted aloe with all the aloin (laxative properties) removed.

164

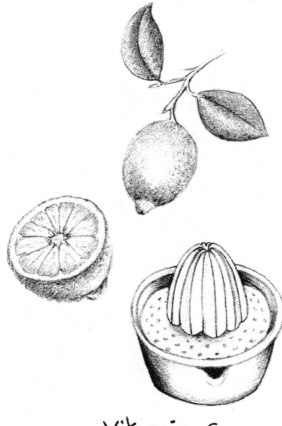

Vitamin C

24

VITAMIN C: THE WONDER NUTRIENT

Hans Larsen states:

Vitamin C was first isolated in 1928 by the Hungarian biochemist and Nobel Prize winner Dr. Syent-Gyorgijc. Vitamin C plays an important role as a component of enzymes involved in the synthesis of collagen and carnitine.

Vitamin C intake markedly reduces the severity of a cold; it also effectively prevents secondary viral and bacterial complications. Vitamin C works by stimulating the immune system and protecting against damage by the

167

free radicals released by the body in its fight against infection. (54)

Drs. Pauling and Cameron pioneered the use of large doses of Vitamin C (more than 10 grams a day) in the treatment of cancer patients. From their experiments at the Vale of Leven Hospital in Scotland, they concluded that terminal cancer patients who received large daily doses of Vitamin C, along with the regular treatment, lived much longer than patients who did not receive Vitamin C. These patients also had less pain, and in general, a much-improved quality of life.

Larsen continues:

> Vitamin C is truly a wonder nutrient and there is no doubt that many of the serious degenerative diseases plaguing the civilized world today can be prevented or even reversed through an adequate intake of this essential vitamin.
>
> A scientific advising panel to the U.S. government recently recommended that all healthy adults increase their Vitamin C intake to 250-1000 mg. a day.
>
> A daily intake of 250-1000 mg. of Vitamin C may be adequate for preventive purposes, but far larger quantities are required in halting or reversing cancer and heart disease and hepatitis C.
>
> Although there has been some concern that people suffering from hemochromatosis (a tendency to iron overload) may be sensitive to high doses of Vitamin C, most researchers

agree that Vitamin C is entirely safe in daily quantities of 10 grams or more. An adequate intake of Vitamin C is surely the best and most cost efficient health insurance available today.

The official Recommended Daily Allowance (RDA) is sixty mg. per day. How much do we need? To answer this question it is crucial to realize that the RDA is not, in any way, based on what is required for optimum health. The RDA is simply the amount required to avoid scurvy, the most obvious deficiency disease. Actually the RDA is based on the Vitamin C content of the average diet. The logic goes somewhat like this: The average "healthy" North American diet provides about 60 mg. per day of Vitamin C, so since scurvy is virtually unknown in the USA today, 60 mg. per day must be adequate. So much for "science."

High-potency Vitamin C produces dramatic healing in many hepatitis C patients. I used C Aspa Scorb by Progressive Laboratories, Inc. It comes in powder form and the dose recommended is one teaspoon, three times a day or approximately fourteen thousand (14,000) mg. This product also contains selenium 270 mcg. You mix a teaspoon full in a small amount of distilled water or juice.

Research papers have reported that RNA viruses, including hepatitis C, encode selenium-dependent glutathione peroxide genes. Research indicates that selenium may act like a "birth control pill" for the virus.

When I first employed Dr. D for my liver problem, his first diagnosis was hemochromatosis. This was, according to him, an inherited disease. He asked if any of my relatives had ever had this disease. Most of my relatives were dead from cancer, so I didn't know.

I experienced a horrendous iron overload in my liver. Chronic hepatitis C does cause iron overload, mostly in male patients, and there are several known adverse effects. I'm sure a lot of unknown problems result from iron overload. That is why Dr. D prescribed phlebotomies or bloodletting for me, in order to leach the iron from my liver. My bloodletting is what led to the blood bank discovering my hepatitis C.

Drinking distilled water helps leach out iron and other toxic overloads from the liver. All chronic hepatitis C patients should drink distilled water during the night.

As long as we're on the topic of iron retention, it is important for hepatitis C patients to avoid all iron supplements. Carefully read the ingredients in supplements because iron is added needlessly in all sorts of pills and other types of supplements such as super-foods and in particular supplements designed for women. If you have hepatitis C and don't know if you're retaining iron in your liver, get tested. A simple blood test will reveal your iron binding content. If you have a liver biopsy, be sure to remind your doctor to have an iron test done at the same time. Not all doctors know or remember to do this. In my case they did do it, but they lost it. I wasn't about to visit Dr. "Pocahontas" a second time.

In order to get enough Vitamin C in my diet, I consumed at least two lemons everyday. They should be fresh and organic. Use them in tea, to marinate meat, in stir-fry, and to make lemonade, lemon honey, and distilled water. Put a slice of lemon in your glass of water; it makes water more exciting. There are live enzymes and bioflavonoids in fresh squeezed fruit that just aren't found in pills, powder, or processed supplements. Also, lemons are a good source of the mineral magnesium, which helps maintain the mineral balance in the body.

Maud Grieve, a modern herbalist said, "It is probable that the lemon is the most valuable of all fruit for preserving health." (55)

Vitamin C leaches calcium out of the body so it is necessary to supplement your body with calcium. Coral Complex, a pure coral from the coral reefs near Japan, has an extra benefit over the standard calcium supplements. Coral Complex aquatic nutrients causes an alkaline balance in the blood. Viruses, tumors and cancers do not like alkaline conditions. There arc also 72 trace minerals in this product as well.

During my treatment I took:

7000 mg. of vitamin C two timcs per day for three months. Vitamin C can leach calcium out of your body. I suggest taking coral calcium with vitamin C as it helps promote an alkaline PH. The vitamin C powder I used contained selenium. Today, I suggest 400 mcgs of selenium per day from all sources.

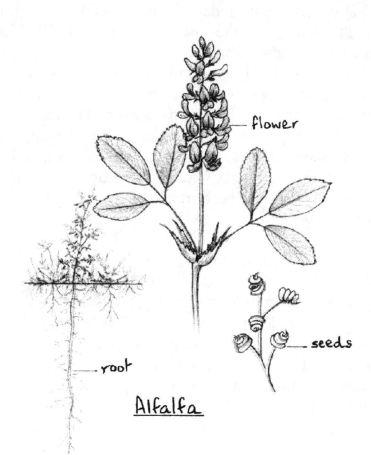

flower

seeds

root

Alfalfa

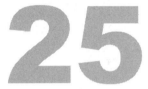

ALFALFA (MEDICAGO SATIVA): THE FATHER OF ALL FOODS

For centuries, alfalfa has been referred to as "the father of all foods." Alfalfa was first cultivated in Persia, and then in 500 B.C., it was then taken to Greece. Alfalfa spread until one day in 1854, it arrived in San Francisco, the American incubator of all good herbs.

Alfalfa has a very unique and distinctive quality that sets it apart from most other plants. The root system of the alfalfa plant reaches thirty feet deep into the soil. This allows the plant to access a large quantity of un-depleted nutrients, salts, and other necessary elements, while most other plants simply don't have this advantage. The leaves of the alfalfa plant contain the eight essential amino acids and ten non-essential amino acids. (Refer to Appendix D for a list of ingredients).

Alfalfa is useful in the treatment of arthritis, urinary tract, kidney and bladder infections, as well as prostate disorders. Alfalfa alkalizes and detoxifies the body, especially the liver.

Studies have shown that alfalfa has inhibited the growth of viruses such as herpes simplex. L-canaverine, a non-protein amino acid, found in alfalfa leaves and roots, has been shown in animal studies to have anti-viral properties and be effective in controlling leukemia and cancer cells.

Alfalfa Leaf Ingredients

Vitamins:	Minerals:	Amino Acids
Beta Carotene	Chromium	Arginine
Vitamin B-1	Calcium	Alanine
Vitamin B-2	Copper	Aspartic Acid
Niacin	Iodine	Cysteine
Vitamin B-6	Iron	Glutamic
Vitamin B-12	Magnesium	Acid
Pantothenic	Acid Manganese	Glycine
Folic Acid	Molybdenum	Histidine
Biotin	Phosphorus	*Isoleucine
P.A.B.A.	Potassium	*Leucine
Inositol	Selenium	*Lysine
Choline*	Sodium	*Methionine
Vitamin C	Zinc	Phenylalanine
Vitamin E		Proline
Vitamin		Serine
(Phylloquinone)		*Threoninc
		Tyrosine
		*Valine

*Denotes an essential amino acid
Pigments: Chlorophyll, Xanthophyll

During my treatment I took:

One gram of alfalfa two times per day.

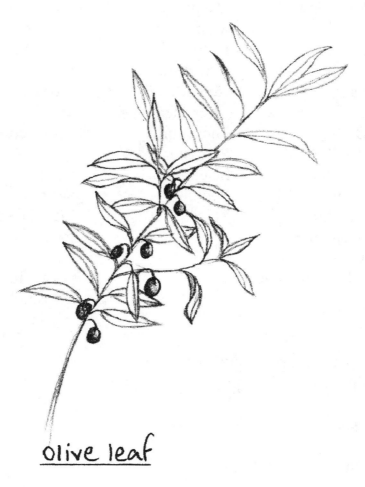

olive leaf

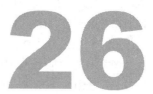

OLIVE LEAF:
NATURE'S ANTIVIRAL

Olive leaf extract is a powerful antiviral and antibacterial agent, and it is also the first botanical mentioned in the Bible: "And the dove came in to him in the evening, and lo, in her mouth was an olive leaf plucked off. So Noah knew that the waters were abated from off the earth." (Genesis 8:11 *King James Bible.)*

A few thousand years later, in Ezekiel 47:12, God speaks of a tree: "The fruit thereof shall be for meat, and the leaf thereof for medicine." Then, in Revelations, at the very end of the *New Testament*, there is an angelic vision of a "tree of life" whose leaves "were for the healing of the nations."

In 1854, the *Pharmaceutical Journal* carried a report by Daniel Hanbury, wherein he said he had discovered olive leaf was an effective tincture and that he had used it successfully in treating his patients in Britain. Dr. Hanbury believed that a bitter substance in the leaves was the key healing ingredient, and he was right. (56)

Many years later, scientists isolated a bitter substance in the olive leaf and named it oleuropein. This chemical is what makes the olive tree resistant to insect and bacterial damage.

Oleuropein is removed from olives when they are cured, so eating olives alone is not going to supply you with this remarkably curative substance.

In 1962, about 100 years later, an Italian researcher reported that ingesting oleuropein lowered blood pressure. Other European researchers confirmed this. They also discovered that olive leaf extract could increase blood flow in coronary arteries, relieve arrhythmias, and prevent intestinal muscle spasms, an important element in treating hepatitis C victims.

A Dutch researcher further determined that the active ingredient in oleuropein is a substance called elenolic acid. In the late 1960s, when drug experimentation was at its best, scientists at Upjohn, a major American pharmaceutical company, demonstrated that elenolic acid inhibited the growth of viruses. In fact, it stopped every virus that it was tested against.

Medical researcher Morton Walker, D.P.M., wrote about olive leaf extract in the July 1996 issue of the *Townsend Letter for Doctors and Patients*: "The intake of flavonoids is correlated with a lower incidence of cardiovascular disease indicating that the daily intake of olive oil and/or olive leaf extract containing phenols will likely bring on a similar result." (57)

According to James R. Privitera, M.D., some of the unique properties of olive leaf are as follows:

- An ability to interfere with critical amino acid production essential for the survival of viruses;
- An ability to contain viral infection and/or spread of it by inactivating the viruses or by preventing virus shedding, budding, or assembly at the cell membrane;
- The ability to directly penetrate infected cells and stop viral replication;
- In the case of retroviruses, olive leaf extract is able to neutralize the production of transcriptase (a protease), which is essential for enabling retroviruses such as HIV to alter the RNA of a healthy cell; and
- It can stimulate phagocytosis, an immune system response in which cells ingest harmful microorganisms and foreign matter (such as bacteria and viruses.) (58)

Olive leaf extract has been shown to be effective against herpes, flu and colds, bacterial infections, diabetes, rheumatoid arthritis, chronic fatigue syndrome, allergies, vaginal yeast infections, skin conditions, malaria, hepatitis B and hepatitis C.

Considering the serious side effects and shortcomings of pharmaceutical drugs, it would be wise to at least try olive leaf for these problems prior to exposing oneself to chemical synthetics.

During my treatment I took:

One 500 mg. of olive leaf extract capsule three days a week.

synapse

dendrites

nucleus

axon

myelin
sheath

node

target
tissue

NADH

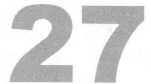

NICOTINAMIDE ADENINE DINUCLEOTIDE (NADH): SYNERGIZE YOUR NEUROTRANSMITTERS

NADH is an incredible supplement, especially for those of you who have undergone the unfortunate use of interferon. One of interferon's best-known side effects is to interfere with the neurotransmissions in the brain stem. In this area of the brain there are approximately fifteen billion brain cells. The messages that come in through your five senses and other important bodily functions are transmitted between these cells by neurotransmitters. Page One of Schiff Supplement Facts reads:

181

NADH is required for synthesis of neurotransmitters, which explains its effects on maintaining healthy mind and mental functions. NADH is the co-enzymatic form of vitamin B-3. NADH is involved in production of energy in all cells.

In my case, interferon devastated these transmissions so much that I could not draw a simple line between numbers on a test given to me by a state-appointed neurologist/psychiatrist. He explained to me that the use of interferon has resulted in symptoms very similar to those of the Gulf War Syndrome.

During and ever since my exposure to that toxic garbage (interferon), my ability to cut a straight line with my skill saw has been eradicated. My once perfect ability as a master carpenter has been erased forever.

NADH is the driving force behind cellular energy production, and it is a very important – if not the most important – antioxidant. It protects your body from free radicals and the ravages of the aging process. It also enhances the capacity of your immune system and protects your cells from damage by toxins and environmental pollution. It increases brain functions and cognitive capabilities. In addition, NADH protects the liver from alcohol damage, prevents the alcohol-induced inhibition of testosterone biosynthesis, normalizes cholesterol levels and blood pressure, and offers protection from certain toxins such as the AIDS drug AZT and other carcinogens without depleting the positive effects of the drug.

NADH is directly involved in the cellular immune defense system. Special white blood cells, called macrophages, are responsible for the direct elimination of foreign bodies, such as bacteria, viruses, and molds. They literally capture these foreign bodies and then degrade and eliminate them. This phenomenon is known as "metabolic burst" and it appears to be the first and most critical step leading to the destruction of foreign invaders.

NADH is present in all living cells. Meat products, fish, and chicken contain the highest amounts. Vegetarian food items contain much less.

Food preparation destroys most NADH and then digestive process destroys even more. Therefore, supplementing with NADH is very helpful in many disease states such as hepatitis C and very important when using "Modern Medicine."

I strongly recommend NADH for all who suffer from hepatitis C. Try it and you'll see why.

During my treatment I took:

Onc 2.5 mg. tablet of NADH each morning on an empty stomach.

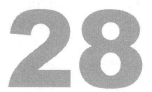

EUROCEL

Eurocel is a product made by Allergy Research Group from herbs that have been used historically in Oriental medicine. (Patrinia villosa, Artemisla capollaris, and Schizandra fructus). After passing chronic and acute toxicity testing in animals, a pilot study was undertaken with HCV patients. The first ten patients reported hepatitis C RNA dropping well below original levels. Further testing is being pursued. The patients were diagnosed positive for antibodies to the hepatitis C virus and showed elevated levels of GPT (glutamic pyruvate transaminase) and had chronic illness for 3 to 20 years before using Eurocel.

Two mg. of the herbal combination were taken twice daily during the study, which lasted from 6 to 24 months. Elevated liver enzyme levels, indicators of liver damage, also dropped to normal levels.

All ten patients in the study showed good response to the herbal application. The prompt reduction of the hepatitis C virus RNA levels gradually lowered during therapy. After 24 months of taking the herbs, the total count of various patients viral titer count decreased from levels in the billions to levels in the thousands, a drop up to one million fold. SGOT (ALT), bilirubin, albumin, total protein, and cholesterol levels were also improved.

Patients reported the following improvements: better quality of sleep, increased physical energy, increased body weight, and smoother, softer skin. This immediate response appeared in the majority of patients. No adverse symptoms were reported.

I suggest two capsules three times per day on an empty stomach.

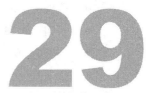

LIPOTROPE

Lipotrope prevents fat accumulation in the liver. The liver removes fatty acids from the diet or from accumulated fat deposits by degrading and oxidizing them when the body must call on fat as a major energy source. Lipotropic factors must be active to prevent abnormal accumulation of fats in the liver. By a process called transmethylation, these lipotropic agents promote the production of lipoproteins, which transfer the fatty acids out of the liver. (62)

Normal liver fat is 5-15%, whereas, a diabetic's liver consists of 25-35% fat. The percentage of liver fat may also be increased by:

- Excessive alcohol consumption
- Birth control pills
- Estrogen usage
- High vitamin B-1 and B12 intake

- Cobalt treatments

Conditions that can result from liver dysfunction include:
- Menstrual irregularities
- Constipation
- Hypertension
- Blood sugar metabolic imbalance
- Fatigue
- Glaucoma
- Arteriosclerosis
- Hepatitis
- Jaundice

Hormone conjugation also occurs in the liver. By keeping the liver healthy, Lipotrope aids in this reaction. Estrogen can be carcinogenic if it is not conjugated. Calcium, protein, mineral, and fat metabolism are all regulated by components of conjugated estrogen. An unhealthy, fatty or cirrhotic liver cannot perform these functions efficiently.

In addition to the protective and regenerative milk thistle herb, Lipotrope includes specific vitamins, minerals, amino acids and herbs, each of which is targeted to lipid metabolism and healthy liver function. These nutrients aid the liver and gallbladder in metabolism of lipids and conjugation of hormones such as estradiol:

Choline is considered one of the B vitamins. It functions with inositol as a basic constituent of lecithin. It appears to be associated primarily with utilization of fats and cholesterol in the body. It prevents fats from accumulating in the liver and facilitates the movement of fats into the cells. Choline combines with fatty acids and phosphoric acid within the liver to form lecithin. It improves liver and gallbladder function and helps prevent gallstones. (63)

Inositol, like choline, is a constituent of lecithin, which is needed to move fats from the liver to the cells. High intake of caffeine may create an inositol shortage in the body. (63)

Vitamin B-6 is involved in the metabolism of fats and fatty acids, especially the essential unsaturated fatty acids. Birth control pills increase the risk of gallstones, which can be caused by oxalic acid toxicity. Vitamin B-6 detoxifies oxalic acid. (67)

Vitamin B-12 and Folic Acid are used in the synthesis of methionine and choline. The coenzyme of vitamin B-12 is a carrier of methyl groups and hydrogen and is necessary for carbohydrate, protein, and fat metabolism. Because of its methyl transfer role, vitamin B-12 is active in the synthesis of the amino acid methionine from its precursor, homocysteine. The coenzyme transfers methyl groups from methyl folate, a derivative of folic acid, to homocysteine and methionine is formed. Because methionine is needed in choline synthesis, B-12 plays a secondary role in the lipid pathway. A choline deficiency that causes fatty liver can be prevented by vitamin B-12 and the other methyl donors: betaine, methionine, and folic acid. (63)

PABA (para-aminobenzoic acid) stimulates the bacteria in the intestines, enabling them to produce folic acid, which in turn aids in the production of pantothenic acid. (63)

Pantothenic Acid has clinical application in lipogenesis formation of cholesterol, formation of steroid hormones and detoxification of drugs. (62)

Magnesium is necessary for coenzyme A reaction. This mineral has been shown to enhance enzymatic activity in the liver. (64) Vitamin and trace mineral deficiencies lower coenzyme activity. (61). In case studies, magnesium has been credited with dissolving gallstones. (67) Alcohol consumption increases the dietary need for magnesium threefold. (64)

Celandine is primarily used as a liver-detoxifying herb for the treatment of hepatitis, jaundice, cancer, psoriasis, eczema, and skin problems. (68)

Chionanthus is a mild stimulant for the bowels and a tonic that strengthens or invigorates organs or the entire organism. This herb has a beneficial effect on the kidneys and liver, including acute and chronic liver inflammation and cirrhosis of the liver. (66) It has been used successfully in treating menstrual disorders, hepatic derangements, jaundice, enlarged spleen and jaundice with arrest of menses. (65)

Black Radish appears to help speed up the flow of bile and has a detoxifying effect on the liver and spleen. (67)

Beet Leaves have been found to increase bile flow as well as aid in carbohydrate and fat metabolism. (67)

Betaine is a source of methyl groups. It is used in the liver for the detoxification of free radicals and other active by-products. (67)

Methionine acts as a methyl donor and antioxidant in liver tissues and aids healing and detoxification of these tissues. (67) Its primary lipotropic function is to prevent excess fat accumulations in the liver by increasing lecithin production. (68)

No specific claim is made for this nutritional preparation. Any recommendations for its use are based solely upon the discretion of the doctor or other qualified medical health care practitioner. This information in this chapter is based upon authoritative and reliable sources.

Lipotrope Formula (per capsule)

Milk Thistle (Silybum marianum)	100 mg.
Choline Bitartrate	150 mg.
Inositol	75 mg.
Vitamin B-6	5 mg.
Vitamin B-12	100 mcg.
Folic Acid	100 mcg.
Pantothenic Acid	125 mg.
PABA	50 mg.
Vitamin C	50 mg.
DI-Methionine	50 mg.
Betaine3HCI	60 mg.
Black Radish	50 mg.
Green Beet Leaf Powder	30 mg.
Chionanthus	30 mg.
Magnesium Aspartate	25 mg.
Celandine (Shelidonium majas)	15 mg.

During my treatment I took:

One to two lipotrope capsules three times per day.

CLEANLINESS AND ALBUMIN

Cleanliness is a key factor in the control and prevention of all disease. In Exodus, Chapter 15:26 we find:

> If thou wilt diligently hearken to the voice of the Lord thy God, and wilt do that which is right in his sight, and wilt give ear to his commandments, and keep all his statutes, I will put none of these diseases upon thee, which I have brought upon the Egyptians: for I am the Lord that healeth thee.

Numbers, Chapter 19:

> And the Lord spoke unto Moses and unto Aaron saying... You can look it up and read it

for yourself. God prescribed detailed methods for using water, various herbs and drying time to cleanse the body properly under several different circumstances: in dealing with the dead, for the prevention of spreading disease, bacteria, viruses and also for the washing of cloths. (Note: Hyssop was the major component referred to.)

McMillan recounts:

In the early 1840's a young doctor named Ignay Semmelweis was given charge over one of the obstetrical wards. He observed that those women who were examined became sick and died much more often than the women who were not examined. After watching this heartbreaking situation for three years, he established a new rule for his ward. He ordered every physician and medical student who had participated in autopsies of the dead to carefully wash his hands before examining living maternity patients.

In April 1847, before the new rule went into effect, fifty-seven (or one out of six) women had died in Dr. Semmelweis's ward. Then he instituted the hand-washing rule. In June, only one out of every forty-two women died. In July, only one out of every eighty-four women died. This is a fourteen-fold decrease in mortality! These astonishing statistics strongly indicated that fatal infections had been carried from corpses to living patients.

One day, after performing autopsies and washing their hands, the physicians and students entered the medical ward and examined a row of beds containing twelve women. Eleven of the twelve women quickly developed temperatures and died.

Another new thought was born in Semmelweis's alert brain: some mysterious element was evidently carried from one living patient to others, and with fatal consequences. Logically, Selmmelweis ordered that everybody wash his hands carefully after examining each living patient. Immediately, howls of protest were raised against the "nuisance" of washing, washing, washing, but as a result the mortality rate went down further.

Was Semmelweis acclaimed by his fellows? To the contrary, lazy students, prejudiced obstetricians, and jealous superiors scorned and belittled him so much that he was dismissed from the hospital. His successor threw out the washbasins and up shot the mortality rate to the old terrifying figures. Were his colleagues convinced then? Not at all. Even the world-renowned pathologist Rudolf Verchow continued to ridicule Semmelweis. We mortals might as well face it – our heads are so hardened by pride and prejudice that proof can rarely penetrate them. (59)

The necessity of hand-washing is a principal that God gave to Moses thirty-five hundred years ago to prevent the spread of disease.

The above-described scenario lends itself to modern medicine's rejection of herbal remedies. Show the doctors the results and they snarl, grin, and make ridiculing comments. Medical doctors are the most brazen pigs on earth.

Doctors throughout history have shunned this principal in part, even when introduced by brilliant experimenting minds. They now accept the fact they must wash their hands frequently.

Albumin is involved in just about everything your body does. According to scientist Kenneth Seeton, a person's albumin count is the prime factor in determining health. (2)

Dr. Richard Gilleman has documented that a low albumin count is connected to heart disease. The balance of albumin should be at least 4.8 grams per liter. The average in the U.S. is 4.1. The average in Japan is 4.6.

That albumin count is connected to cleanliness – which is next to godliness - is a proven fact. However, every single medical doctor I have mentioned this to has come back with an arrogant response, in particular the "great hepatologist." Upon suggesting to him the connection between an individual's albumin count and wellness, his response in part was "that is the most ridiculous thing I've heard."

The thinking mind aligns the events of history with the words spoken by God and with seemingly new discoveries and then connects them.

I here and now inform you that the majority of people who are mentally equipped to become doctors, for the most part, are so head strong and resistant to reality that they reside only in the cubical of education they received or are required to take.

The problem lies in the field. It's like a farmer. If he owns a field, he farms it. He doesn't cross over and farm something that isn't his. Doctors are indoctrinated in their learned behavior and allow in little else. History proves it, and the FDA is a prime example of this lunacy.

Harmless herbs are considered an expensive sewer additive by the most renowned doctors in the field of hepatitis C. I'm sure that in just a few years these relics of the past will be regarded as fools of a dark age.

Kenneth Seeton also introduces the challenge that there are two minds: the mind of the immune system and the mind of the brain. When the immune system is overloaded, it robs the ability of the mind to develop or function at full capacity, thus robbing you of your full IQ potential. If your antibody measure is being lowered to support your immune system defense, you have less for intellectual development. In order to have a higher IQ, you need a purified brain, which results if you remove the overload on the immune system. One way to lower the overload is to wash your hands and fingernails with an antibiotic, four to twenty times a day.

The need for cleanliness brings us to the conclusion that Moses was more correct than we ever thought possible and it's all very scientific. For those of you who don't believe, consider this: God is real.

Kenneth Seeton believes that eighty percent of all disease is transmitted through rubbing of the eyes and nose. Self-inoculated fingertips are the most effective way to transmit ear, nose and throat problems.

The albumin count cannot be raised by diet. The only way to bring the antibodies down is by removing the possibility of infection from eyes and nose. To look at this in a more convincing way, consider the fact that one gram of albumin equals twelve trillion molecules.

If you wish to overcome hepatitis C, it is critical to follow the previous scenario absolutely in order to free up the immune system and boost it in order to conquer your potentially fatal disease.

Remember, "You can't create Shakespeare in a dirty house." The relation of albumin to health and cleanliness "is the largest discovery in medical history." (60)

I suggest that we consider conventional medicine to be in transition, rather than factual, which is what the greatest alternative doctors gave to me.

We need to transition back to God as our good shepherd, who created everything and told us how to deal with all things. We have simply failed at studying, understanding and practicing His word.

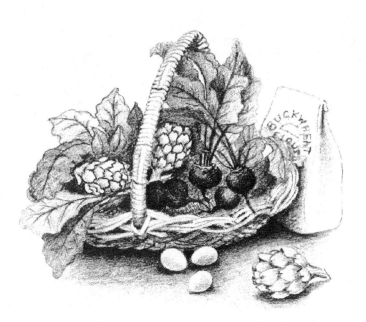

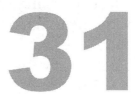

FOODS FOR HEALTH

Artichokes (Cynara Scolymus L.) "Two Artichokes A Day Keeps the Doctor Away."

Artichokes are a native of the Mediterranean and a perennial in the thistle group, the same group as milk thistle. Dr. Finnegan prescribed two artichokes per day, preferably organically grown. I suggest you wash them thoroughly. The organic ones often have bugs, while the non-organic ones have insecticides. Many people feel that artichokes are too labor intensive. Be assured they are well worth the effort.

Artichokes also can be obtained marinated or plain in jars and cans. A typical can of artichoke hearts ranges in cost from $1.99 to $4.00. They make a great appetizer and are good in salads. If you like deep fried foods, batter them up, dump them in some good oil (like olive), and they are the best.

There is also a company named De Boles that produces pastas of all types made from the Jerusalem artichoke flower. They have macaroni and cheese, spaghetti, linguine, lasagna, and all shapes and sizes of pasta. You can – and should – literally inundate your diet with every sort of artichoke as much as possible. These products love your liver. They possess properties that clean and help restore liver function.

Jean Carper found:

A series of studies in 1940 by a Japanese researcher found that the artichoke lowered total cholesterol somewhat, stimulated production of bile by the liver, performed as a diuretic, and enhanced 'well-being strikingly'.

In 1969, French scientists were so successful in using artichoke extract for treating liver and kidney ailments that they took out a patent on it. In fact, cynarin, a constituent of the artichoke, was formulated into a drug lowering blood cholesterol. Cynarin also is well known to be liver protective. (69)

Distilled Water

It is important that the hepatitis C patient consume more than an average amount of water frequently throughout the day and night. I suggest that you keep a bottle of distilled water next to your bed and drink some each time you wake up during the night. This helps cleanse the liver by removing toxins and other unwanted substances. Drink your favorite water during the day.

Raw Eggs

Eat one raw egg per day. They are easy to digest and contain many enzymes and live food source nutrients that cooked eggs simply don't have. They are great in milk shakes or pop one in your colostrum drink. Raw eggs are best in orange juice. Drop one in a blender, pour in 6-8 ounces of fresh organic orange juice and blend. You can also add some "Pure Synergy," progreens, or your favorite green food product. For an extra treat, after blending add some sparkling water and stir lightly. This is a terrific way to start the day.

Jean Carper continues:

Chickens have lots of rotavirus infections and the antigen - the viral agent that provides the pattern for the antibody – is similar to that of humans.

Dr. Yolken sees chickens as a virtual antibody factory. He notes that a single chicken could provide up to thirty kilograms of immunoglobin a year. Eggs have the potential of providing a large, economical supply of antibodies, fit for consumption by all ages.

Buckwheat

Buckwheat has been widely recognized as a great

cleanser for the liver. You can incorporate it into pancakes instead of flour or wherever flour is needed. Also, you can find cereals and noodles made from buckwheat in many health food stores.

Spinach

Spinach is prescribed as a preventive against hepatocellular carcinoma. Even though spinach is rich in iron, and we want to avoid iron, much of the iron in spinach is not absorbed because it is inside a cell membrane. This cell membrane often doesn't break down, and therefore passes through your system.

Several studies have indicated there are properties in spinach that help to prevent liver cancer.

Jean Carper found:

> A new United States Department of Agriculture analysis finds that raw spinach has thirty-six milligrams of total arotenoids per hundred grams; whereas raw carrots have fourteen milligrams per hundred grams, most of it in beta-carotene. Although beta-carotene is a confirmed cancer antagonist, spinach's panoply of other carotenoids may possess anti-cancer activity,· and may be even more responsible than beta-carotene for spinach's splendid showing in population surveys of cancer-preventive foods.

Foods that are good for liver function:

Foods that are especially good for rebuilding the liver are: hemp seeds, hemp seed oil, beet tops, beets, artichokes, lemon juice, carrots, greens, whole grains, and raw yogurt from good quality milk, organic liver, and egg yolks.

The hepatitis C patient needs to recognize that it is easy to overload on protein and soon your ammonia level will start going up. That can get you in big trouble in terms of your central nervous system.

The few doctors who recommend a diet for there hepatitis C patients suggest the elimination of all fried foods, red meat, alcohol, and coffee, while emphasizing cooked vegetables and grains along with limited amounts of chicken, fish, and turkey.

Yogurt: The Super-Immune Booster.

I consumed yogurt daily during my recovery period, and still do. There are many wonderful properties about yogurt that I had no knowledge of. The following are some of them.

Dr. Khem Shahani found:

> Lactobacillus acidophilus DDS-, enhance immune function by eliminating or inhibiting the formation of cancer-causing chemicals. Nitrates, commonly used in food processing, can be converted via enzymes to carcinogenic nitrosamines in the gut. Lactobacillus acidophilus is able to halt this process first by reducing the quantity of potential carcinogens, and second by deactivating certain cancer-causing enzymes, especially d-glucrondase and b-glucosidase.
> The "Benefits of Yogurt," a report published in the *Journal of Immunotherapy,* found that

acidophilus containing yogurt eaten over several months increased gamma-interferon, an important immune-enhancing protein that prevents viruses from reproducing. Also noted was a reduction in inflammatory responses of the gut. IgE, an immunoglobulin that is effective in destroying parasites, is enhanced when lactobacillus bulgaricus was added to the diet. It was found to have powerful antibacterial properties, allowing IgE to function optimally. (70)

Avocados

Researchers in Japan have discovered that avocados contain potent chemicals that may reduce liver damage.

Five compounds appear to be active in reducing liver damage. Each was tested in rats with chemically induced liver injuries. The injuries resembled those caused by viruses, suggesting that avocados may be especially promising for the treatment of viral hepatitis according to the "International Chemical Congress of Pacific Basin Societies."

I created and lived on an avocado farm from 1980 until 1987. During this time, I consumed many avocados. I still do and I suggest you do the same. Enjoy them in salads, sandwiches, guacamole or plain. They taste good, and they are good for your liver.

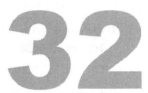

THINGS TO AVOID

Homogenized, Pasteurized Dairy Products

Pasteurization of milk is simply the heating of milk to a high temperature for a period of time to kill certain bacteria. This heating proccss also destroys most of the essential elements of milk, basically making it relatively worthless to consume. You may have noticed that cooked milk often states on the side of the container that the producer has added vitamin D3 and vitamin A. Milk is produced by mothers for the nourishment of their young. This milk contains many essential nutrients, enzymes, and other factors that are destroyed by heat.

Dr. Kurt Oster and many others consider homogenized milk to be the number one cause of heart disease in the United States. (71)

For those of you who weren't raised on a farm, I will attempt to explain why Americans homogenize milk.

In raw milk the butterfat rises to the top of the milk. This amount of butterfat is just too much for the average American to deal with, so along came the process of homogenization. Put simply, homogenization combines the milk and the butterfat. Butterfat is surrounded by a special enzyme that aids in its digestion. This enzyme is known by the initials "X.O." which stands for xanthine oxidase.

Due to the results of homogenization, digestion of raw milk in the stomach barely begins. Most of the fat digestion doesn't really start until in the upper intestine, and it finishes in the liver. The liver is made to handle the digestion and use of fat in our body.

If you drink raw milk, the butterfat with the X.O. enzyme goes into the stomach, then into the small intestine, and finally into the liver. The liver breaks up the fat into what are called fatty acids, and the body uses them. When milk is homogenized, the butterfat is so small that is gets into the stomach and goes into the upper intestine. The butterfat molecules are so small that they can pass right through the upper intestine and directly into your cells.

> However, as this little particle of fat gets into your bloodstream, it will eventually go through the liver and get digested... Due to the liver being a filter, all the blood goes through the liver and gets cleaned. (71)

This process of homogenization causes an impaired liver to work harder to deal with this processed food. It is a completely unnatural food that the human body has never had to deal with until the twentieth century. Beyond stressing the impaired liver:

> The homogenized fat gets into the bloodstream; it carries along with it the XO enzyme. Once the XO enzyme gets inside of an artery, it eats and attacks the inside of the artery wall. (71)

This doesn't just happen in milk. It happens with everything made from milk; cottage cheese, cheese, and sour cream, etc. Luckily we can now purchase raw milk and raw milk products in many states.

When I was a small boy, I used to help my father milk the cows. He would pour the pails of milk into a red contraption called a separator. I would turn the large red handle and out one spout would come cream, and out of the other, fat-free raw milk. We would then churn the cream into butter in a large round wooden cylinder with a stick coming out the top. We even made real ice cream with fresh, raw cream from cows that never thought of eating chicken manure or who had ever had a hormone shot. It sure tasted better than anything I can remember.

Considering the quality of the milk available in the modern world, you might consider supplementing with Colostrum, which is milk taken from a mammal, usually cows, from the time they give birth until approximately 18 hours later. This milk is filled with many wonder-nutrients that are simply not found elsewhere. Colostrum is an essential immune booster.

Hard Liquor

Liquor is hard on your liver. The best reason I can think of not to drink liquor is because if you are a drinker, the probability of receiving a liver transplant – if you ever need one – is slim to none. Also, consumption of large amounts of alcohol inflames the liver and for people with hepatitis C, it usually makes you feel sicker, which takes the fun out of it. It is best to minimize your alcohol intake or better yet do away with it all together.

Sugar Substitutes (Saccharine, Equal, etc.)

It is my understanding that sugar substitutes, especially saccharine, require sixty times more effort by the liver to process than sugar. Also, I suggest that the next time you go out to eat and see one of those little pink packages on the table, pick it up and read the back. It says in plain English, "This product has been shown to cause cancer…" Use honey and raw sugar instead.

Analysis shows nearly 100% of independent research finds problems with aspartame (NutraSweet). Findings issued by the Aspartame Toxicity Information Center in 1996 stated:

> An analysis of peer reviewed medical literature using MEDLINE and other databases was conducted by Ralph G. Walton, MD, Chairman, The Center for Behavioral Medicine, Professor of Clinical Psychiatry, Northeastern Ohio Universities College of Medicine. Dr. Walton analyzed 162 studies that were felt to have relevance to the human safety question. Of those studies, 74 studies had aspartame Industry-sponsorship and 90 were funded without any industry money.

Of the 90 non-industry-sponsored studies, 83 (92%) identified one or more problems with aspartame. Of the 7 studies that did not find a problem, 6 of those studies were conducted by the FDA. Given that a number of FDA officials went to work for the aspartame industry immediately following approval (including the former FDA Commissioner), many consider these studies to be equivalent to industry-sponsored research.

Of the 74 aspartame industry-sponsored studies, all 74 (100%) claimed that no problems were found with aspartame. This is reminiscent of tobacco industry research where it is primarily the tobacco research that never finds problems with the product, but nearly all of the independent studies do find problems.

The seventy-four aspartame industry industry-sponsored studies are those, which one invariably sees cited in PR/news reports and reported by organizations funded by Monsanto/Benevia/NutraSweet (e.g., IFIC, ADA). These studies have serve design deficiencies which help guarantee the "desired" outcomes. (72)

Medical Doctors

The people who attach M.D. to their name should be avoided completely during your healing process. Hopefully, after reading this book, you can understand why I feel the way I do. If, for some reason you cannot, here are a few more reasons. They are very expensive, and they know nothing about curing hepatitis C. They do know how to prescribe interferon, but you don't want to take interferon except as a last resort. Finally, if you get to the point of a liver transplant, then of course, medical doctors are the only resource. I only hope you pick one who is a good mechanic and who has a good supply of livers.

In a blistering report released on November 29, 1999, a prestigious medical group said America's entire health care system needs "dramatic changes" to cut the enormous number of deaths and injuries from medical errors. (3)

This Group said hospitals should report mistakes to the federal government, not keep them secret as they often do now.

Dr. Sid Wolfe of Public Citizen, a consumer watchdog group, said:

> Medical errors in hospitals and elsewhere have been buried for too long, and it is long overdue that they need to be reported to public agencies. (73)

Experts say between 44,000 and 98,000 Americans die from mistakes every year in hospitals alone. That makes hospital errors the eighth leading cause of death – actually ahead of traffic accidents, breast cancer and AIDS.

The report from the Institute of Medicine, a division of the National Academy of Sciences, said the numbers could be cut sharply. It sets as "a minimum goal a 50 percent reduction in errors over five years."

Attorney Andrew Meyer said:

The medical profession seems to like to keep the errors that are made a secret in order to maintain the faith in the profession. (74)

This article was reported on the front page of *USA Today*, the *Washington Post* and *The New York Times*. The *L A Times* refers to the story on page 3.

How many occupations do you know of that can kill 98,000 people a year and not have it hit the headlines for decades? This statistic, 98,000, is just short of DOUBLE the number of Americans killed in Vietnam. (For additional information on medical doctors refer to Addendum 2).

Hydrogenated Oil

Dr. John Finnegan warns:

More than 200 million people may have been killed by refined oils. More people may have been killed from the harmful effects of refined oils and the deficiency of Omega-3 fatty acids than have been killed by all the wars of the century.

Many people are greatly concerned about the continuing increase in degenerative disease today. They understand that there is a connection between our consumption of refined and hydrogenated oils – including those contained in margarine and many processed foods – and the breakdown of our health and immune systems. (75)

It is nearly impossible to buy a cookie, cracker, cake, cereal, bread, donut, or pastry (and the list goes on) that does not contain hydrogenated oil. Dr. Ed Wagner told me that it could take six to nine months for hydrogenated oil to pass through the liver, thus acting as a literal poison.

Stress

It is hard to avoid stress, especially when your doctor has just announced that you have hepatitis C and you are going to die a horrible death. You give up the idea of ever receiving a liver transplant when he tells you that forty people die waiting for a liver transplant for every one who gets one. Then he says "imagine yourself well, but also make sure your will is in order." He sends you on your way with a prescription for interferon, which will no doubt cause you to beat your mate, hate your children, and kill your dogs. Stress may seem minor compared to being subjected to this scenario, which I can tell you is not exaggerated.

Livers don't like stress. So buy a lotto ticket and dream at least a few minutes a day, just to escape reality for a little while. The body is not designed to deal with stress for more than short periods of time. Stress breaks down the immune system and that's what we want to boost. Read my book again and again, that should greatly relieve stress. Consult a spiritual advisor. Enjoy life!

Prayer is good, and it works. Consult your pastor and have your church include you in the intercessory prayer meetings.

Take time out from your schedule and do something you don't usually do. If you like Bob Dylan, go to a Dylan concert.

EAT CHOCOLATE! Chocolate is a mild mood elevator and a good antioxidant.

DURING MY TREATMENT I TOOK:

- Two 200 mg. organic *Milk Thistle* capsules three times per day. I also drank one quart of milk thistle tea per day.
- One vial of *Natcell Thymus* on an empty stomach every other day for 18 months. I also took two 500 mg. of thymus organic capsules three times per day.
- One 300 mg. *Adrenal* organic capsule two times per day. I suggest taking *Natcell Adrenal*, one vial per week (optional).
- Two 500 mg. *Liver* organic capsules two times per day. I suggest taking *Natcell Liver*, two vials per week (optional).
- Two cups of *Reishi* tea per day. You may also take Reishi capsules; one 500 mg. three times per day.
- Two 100 mg. *Lipoic Acid* capsules two times per day. Today, I suggest taking one 200 mg. lipoic acid capsule three times per day.
- One 500 mg. *Licorice Root* capsule two times per day, five days a week. I also drank two cups of licorice tea five days a week.
- One 500 mg. organic *Dandelion Root* capsule three times per day. I also drank one quart of dandelion root tea every evening.
- Two 500 mg. *Cat's Claw* capsules two times per day. I also drank two cups of cat's claw tea per day.
- Four oz. of properly prepared *Aloe Vera* two to four times per day, usually more.
- 7000 mg. of *Vitamin C* two times per day for three months. Vitamin C can leach calcium out of your body. I suggest taking coral calcium with vitamin C as it helps promote an alkaline PH.

- One 200 mcg. *Selenium* capsule two times per day.
- One gram of *Alfalfa* two times per day.
- One 2.5 mg. tablet of *NADH* each morning on an empty stomach.
- Two capsules of *Eurocel* (alternative to Hepastat) three times per day on an empty stomach.
- One to two *Lipotrope (*same as Hepata Trope) capsules three times per day.

OTHER BENEFICIAL SUPPLEMENTS:

- *Vitamin B Complex* - one capsule three times per day.
- *MSM* - for many types of arthritis and joint pain caused by hepatitis C.
- *Flax Seed Oil* - Alpha-Linolenic Acid, Omega-3, 6 and 9.
- *COQ10 -* oxygenates the blood.
- *Natcell Pancreas* - helps with blood sugar problems, Type II Diabetes, cancer.
- *Natcell Mesenchyme* - the fluid in the embryo that gives rise to all organs.

HERB SCHEDULE 1

--TAKE AFTER WAKING UP, ON AN EMPTY STOMACH--							
NATCELL	Mon	Tue	Wed	Thurs	Fri	Sat	Sun
THYMUS	X		X		X		X
LIVER		X				X	
ADRENAL				X			
MESENCHYME		X			X		
PANCREAS	Depends on condition						

VITAMIN C	To tolerance
ALOE JUICE	4 oz. 3 times per day or more
MILK THISTLE TEA	Several cups per day
DANDELION TEA	1 quart per day: late afternoon and evening
REISHI TEA	2 cups per day
LICORICE TEA	2 cups per day
HYSSOP TEA	(fast) 2 quarts per day for 3 days, once a month
PURE SYNERGY	Mix with orange juice and one raw egg per day
PROGREENS	One scoop per day
RAW EGG	One per day, can use with Pure Synergy
ARTICHOKE	1-2 per day
BUCKWHEAT	Pancakes, bread, noodles – use instead of flour

HERB SCHEDULE 2

	Empty Stomach	Breakfast	Lunch	Dinner
ALFALFA	X	2 tablets, 2 times a day		
NADH	X	1 (2.5mg) tablet per day		
EUROCEL	X	2 caps, 2 times a day		
MODUCARE	X	1-2 caps, 3 times a day		
ADRENAL		2	1	
CATS CLAW			500mg	
DANDELION		560mg	560mg	560mg
MILK THISTLE		400mg	400mg	400mg
LIPOTROPE		1	1	1
LIPOIC ACID		200mg	200mg	200mg
IMMUNO GLAND		1	1	1
LICORICE			1	1
LIVER		500mg	500mg	500mg
THYMUS		1000mg	1000mg	1000mg
REISHI		500mg	500mg	500mg
ARTICHOL PRO		1	1	1
VITAMIN B			1	1
CORAL COMPLEX		1	1	1
OLIVE LEAF			1	1
M.G.N.3		Varies according to condition		
COLOSTRUM		Varies according to type		
PANCREAS		Varies according to condition		
SELENIUM		400 mcgs per day from all sources		

There are some items listed not covered in this book. These are items that have shown promise in the treatment of hepatitis C. For a complete description, go to www.hepatitiscfree.com.

TAKE ACTION NOW!
LETTERS FROM SURVIVORS
AND THOSE WHO PRACTICED
MODERN MEDICINE

Hepatitis C is a life-threatening virus, but doctors are still treating hepatitis C patients with interferon, even though this "therapy" and all its combinations have proven to be a complete failure. Rather than recognizing the value of natural therapies, they recommend to thousands of patients that they simply wait for a liver transplant. Many die waiting. Many more die from other complications from hepatitis C, which a liver transplant cannot help.

Fortunately, in the 21st century, man has re-discovered time-proven natural healing. As a culture, we are becoming more aware of the fact that we can support our immune systems and help them achieve what they do best – heal.

I believe that with knowledge and persistence we can achieve optimum health. Unfortunately it takes time, money, and sacrifice to learn about and acquire the necessary natural herbal supplements, but you can't wait!

The following is feedback I have gotten from my readers. I hope that these testimonials will inspire hope in hepatitis C sufferers and instill in them the determination necessary for their survival.

The first letter is from Debra Caprianos who writes about her husband's struggle with hepatitis C. It makes the point that time is of the essence. Don't waste your time worrying about money. Instead, use your time to make more time. Take action now. Read on:

May 25, 2000

Dear Lloyd,

Regarding my telephone conversations with you in recent days, I can't begin to tell you how much your kindness and compassion means to me. Your sharing of information as to what I could do to possibly help my husband while he was in the hospital was sincerely appreciated. It's nice to know that among the human population there are pockets of truly good, kind, and selfless individuals striving to help others without the obvious ulterior motives (and we know what those are). You are an angel!

My husband passed away last Wednesday. During the last week of his life my frantic research led me to four different methods of helping his condition, one of which was yours, and all the people involved with these methods were the kindest of individuals. I felt blessed having made their acquaintance. But unfortunately it was too little – too late. My husband lingered in the hospital for four weeks and so did I. The nurses managed to scrape up a cot for me, and as I slept there each night by his bed, time became irrelevant.

My daughter, who is 21, came up with the idea of having an alternative funeral service for him, which I wholeheartedly supported. I've been a "truth-seeker" pursuing the spiritual path for 20 years now, and my daughter Jamie is following a similar course (though she's far wiser at her age than I ever was; I find many of the young are further ahead in wisdom than many adults ever were at their age). So we put together a beautiful service, which we referred to not as a funeral, but a "rebirth celebration."

This was very appropriate since my husband gave the most treasured gifts of all to my children and me. You must understand here that he was a man of few words, incredibly strong, never complained when he felt pain, and a businessman to boot, a type A personality. The only time he verbally rattled on was when it involved speaking about his audio/visual business. As for spirituality and such as seeing through the "veil of illusion" (I remembered you liked that expression), it was another world for him. But when he went into his first coma on Good Friday, my daughter and I prayed, hoping to bring him back to consciousness and healing. Well, Easter Sunday he regained his consciousness. The following day Jamie asked her father very casually what he had experienced during his coma. He looked into her eyes, pulled the covers up around his neck, and said very seriously, "Jamie I know this might sound crazy but it's true what they say. In a flash I found myself in the most beautiful magical world you could ever imagine. I was dancing and playing and singing. I have never felt so free and happy in all my life. It was soooo beautiful." She then asked if he had seen a white light and he replied, "Oh yes the white light was there, but it was unlike any white light you could ever imagine in this physical world." She then asked if he had a choice to come back and he said, "Yes, I did have a choice but I was enjoying myself so much that I really didn't want to come back. But eventually everything started to fade, and here I am." Apparently he confided in her that he had many such experiences, but he could only remember this one to tell her at that time. This was the gift he gave us; he let us know that his passing didn't mean he was fading off into some oblivion or deep, dark hole. It was the absolute knowing that he has passed on to some wonderful, happy, magical world, a world he expressed to Jamie as being "better than Disney world." This truly comforts us during our terrible times of missing him. No amount of money could put a price on this gift.

The guests were informed not to come in black, but to wear lighter colors, and we incorporated nature into the service to emphasize the cycle of rebirth. We had wonderful feedback from all who attended that it was the most beautiful "funeral" they had ever attended. In every respect, it was truly a celebration of who he was and a celebration of life, which is something he always wished to do, live, but hepatitis C deprived him of his life.

But just the same, with him gone now, I feel as if I've been jettisoned into the *Twilight Zone* – one moment they're here and the next they're gone forever.

Lloyd, thank you so much for your book and all of the photocopies! I received them in the mail yesterday and have begun to read the book. Fabulous! I can feel your heart and soul in it! What a nightmare you experienced; it makes me understand so much more of what excruciating hell my husband experienced all those years without ever letting me know the full truth of what was happening to him. His determination to protect his wife and children was a destructive, misinformed obsession.

Understanding what torture you experienced made me understand why in those days before he entered the hospital it was as if I were looking into the eyes of a drowning man. He was literally drowning in his own bodily fluids. The lymphatic fluids that had been accumulating in his body over the last several years had been mistaken for body fat. His legs became so waterlogged that he could barely walk and his penis disappeared into his pubic area somewhere. The poor man was at his wits end wondering why his thighs and legs kept ballooning. He had constant abscesses between his thighs that would break open and bleed. His problems were numerous. It was hell for me, because subconsciously I knew he was a dying man (looking into his eyes was torture), but I couldn't figure out what was wrong. I believe he was quite confused himself, in spite of the fact that he knew he had hepatitis C. He had a list of more than a dozen doctors he'd been seeing. Goodness knows what they told him. It's all guesswork for me now. But suffer, did he ever!

I intend at some point to get in touch with you again because I would like to share your book with hepatitis C patients here in Toronto. So when my life and finances are in order, I will order several copies to give to those looking for the kind of help you offer. I will mention your name whenever I can. You deserve it! I'll need time to come to terms with this new direction in my life, but when I'm back on top of things, I'll connect again.

Thanks for being the champion you are! We need brave men like you, there are far too few in the world today!

Yours truly,
Debra Capranos

Everyday I hear stories from victims of hepatitis C that would be easily dismissed as fiction by the medical community not to mention the average American. With their arrogant attitudes and demeaning behavior, many doctors just smile and chuckle when asked about the healing potential of herbs. However, some of the success stories I've heard from my clients can't just be dismissed with a chuckle and a smile. In fact, a good number of their stories are even more dramatic than my own personal account.

For example, today I heard from a client of mine in Arizona. She's forty-two years old and only three months ago she underwent gallbladder surgery. She had a liver biopsy performed during the procedure. The results of the biopsy were clear: chronic hepatitis C, stage 2 cirrhosis. Her hepatologist told her that her condition was too bad to treat with interferon and that she would need a liver transplant. He put her on the list.

After some research, the woman read this book (*Triumph Over Hepatitis C.*, 1st Edition). Liking what she saw, she decided to give the program a try. After three months on the program, she returned to see the doctor at the University of Arizona Teaching Hospital. Upon seeing her, the doctor admits he did not expect to see her looking so healthy.

When she told the doctor that she had been taking herbs, he immediately stated, "I must have been wrong; I must have made a mistake when I read your reports." Her retort was, "LISTEN to me; I've been taking herbs!"

Ignoring her, the doctor handed her a form to sign so he could acquire the slides of her biopsy to re-examine them. Then he made the statement, "You cannot get well from this condition."

I would love to meet this "fool" in a public forum and debate these issues with him.

Recently another terrific story unfolded. A forty-year-old female called me. She sounded like she was near death: weak, confused, hopeless, and definitely older than her actual years. She told me that following my program cured her friend. She said she was reading my book and that she needed my help because her doctor was killing her. She told me about the horrors she had faced. Her doctor has had her on interferon since 1997 – that's 11 months on, 2 months off, 11 months on, two months off for four years.

I told her with a drug protocol like this that she should already be dead. Then she told me she has been on pegulated interferon for 5 weeks. We talked for a couple of hours during which time she told me more about how terrible her life has been and her husband confirmed her troubles. She told me she has had 4 liver biopsies. When she read them to me, I thought to myself, "these are the best liver biopsies I've ever heard." Then she told me that her doctor told her that her viral load was off the charts, that it was so high it couldn't be counted! The test she was given was PCR RNA HCV Qualitative, the test with a range that just states, "greater than 850,000."

It seemed to me that she was being used as a guinea pig in order to determine the long-term effects of interferon. I know that not many people could tolerate interferon for that length of time. She was the perfect victim, because of the simple fact that she did not suffer the usual hard effects of interferon.

Then she told me she had pleaded with the doctor to let her stop the pegulated interferon, but he had told her that she would die if she stopped.

I pleaded with her and her husband to stop this insidious criminal activity being perpetuated by her doctor. She agreed, stopped taking interferon, and went on my full program. After a few days, her husband called me late at night and asked, "What have you done to my wife?" He told me that when he came home from work, he found the house clean, cleaner than it had been since his wife had begun taking interferon. He said his wife had also taken down and washed all of the curtains. He happily told me that he and his wife spent the rest of the evening putting the curtains back up. He had his wife back, and I could feel his joy.

How long will it take before conventional medicine realizes that the health of their patients is more important than the money that finds its way into their overstuffed wallets and the bank accounts of the pharmaceutical companies? Hopefully, not too long.

The following are just a few of the thousands of letters I've received from people suffering with hepatitis C:

MESSAGE FROM A SURVIVOR:
90% decrease in viral load!

This is to all of you suffering with hepatitis C, especially those of you whose progress in recovery is slow. I was diagnosed with hep C in February of 1999, and considering that I had a friend who had just completed 18 months of pure hell on interferon, I told my doctor that unless he said I would be dead in 5 years without it, I wanted to try to find a better way. Luckily he agreed with me. Referring to interferon he said, "It's nasty stuff."

At this time, my liver enzymes were elevated and my viral load was 62,620,000. I had sold my business of seven years because I was very sick. I started taking some herbs and supplements, and by October of 1999 my viral load was 39,610,000, and I was feeling a bit better. So I slacked off on the herbs. By February of 2000, I was back up to 66,710,000, and I felt like I was dying. So once again, I began taking more herbs.

By September, I had found Lloyd Wright's web site on the Internet, and I had finally gotten it through my thick skull that there really was something to the herbs. I began taking as many of Lloyd's products as I could, and I noticed a dramatic increase in my energy level. Also, my liver stopped aching, my skin stopped itching, and in time, virtually all of my symptoms either went away or diminished tremendously.

I have really struggled from time to time with taking everything like I'm supposed to and with wanting to just give up and die. (I'm only 47 years old.) It's a struggle to discontinue my bad habits and eat healthier. All along the way, Lloyd has encouraged me to keep at it and remember that I had an extremely high viral load and was very sick, so it might take longer for me to recover. I had my blood tested the other day and my liver enzymes are fine. Best of all, my viral load is (are you ready for this?) 6,287,740, which is about a 90% decrease! I am thrilled and so encouraged. I want to get rid of this virus, and I believe I will. It's all up to me. I am the only one who can get up in the morning, go to the freezer, and take out that little brown vial. I am the only one who can make those time-consuming, all-important teas and swallow all those pills all day long. I decided in the very beginning to take matters into my own hands, but sometimes it's very difficult to have the discipline to keep at it. One time I complained to my Doctor about how hard it was to take all this stuff, and he reminded me of the alternatives. He is as supportive as an

MD can be. He also told me that he'd love to have something else to offer his hep C patients (besides combo therapy) and that he'll be real interested to see what happens with me.

When he gave me the results of my viral titer the other day, he told me that it will not be medically significant until it's under 2,000,000. "That's when people respond more favorably to interferon," he said. But that is not why I am doing this, and a 90% decrease is VERY significant to me.

I hope my progress will inspire others to keep at it, be patient, and give it time. I look at this much the same way as I do fertilizers. If you use chemical products, you will get pretty fast results–a green lawn in 2 days–but it doesn't last. It's only cosmetic, and you have to keep doing it over and over. If you use organic products, it will take longer to get the desired result, but you will end up not only with a healthier, greener lawn, you'll also have a healthy root system, without putting deadly chemicals into the environment. It's not a quick fix; it's a process that takes time and patience. I do believe now that all good things come to those who wait.

Sincerely,
Jane

Note from Lloyd:

Jane's e-mails are posted on my website describing how she suddenly found herself doing things instead of lying on the couch all day. People noticed the color was back in her face, and she found that she was singing again. I would like to mention that several months after her viral load dropped from 62,620,000 to 32,000,000, she went in for new tests. She anxiously waited for her test results, and when they came back, she saw she had received the usual "greater than 850,000" test, which is basically worthless. This happened to her a few times in a row and she found it very depressing.

Finally, after about 6 months on my program, her test results came back to 30,000,000. I strongly advised her to begin a new effort to drink the recommended teas and take the new liquid ascorbic C, because the person who created this supplement told me it was designed to enter the blood stream similarly to that of an IV drop. Normally oral vitamin C is only 10% absorbed. Those are the only changes we made and she dropped from 30 million to 6,287,740. This is a terrific response.

Her doctor did not consider her progress "significant." What do you think?

Here is another letter describing success with natural, alternative remedies:

February 2002
Dear Lloyd,

I received my diagnosis early last November 2001, and immediately began to research the disease and my options. I quickly uncovered the truth about interferon as well as the availability of alternative therapies. I soon began a regimen of supplements and kept adding to them as I discovered more information. On November 28th, I received my first set of numbers, plus genotype. My viral load was 628,789 and an ATL of 51.

I kept researching, along with the tireless help of my beautiful wife, and asked for another set of tests before my scheduled appointment with a specialist. My next set of tests was taken on January 2, 2002, and they showed an increased viral load of 815,789 and an ATL of 51. My specialist suggested I have an iron-binding test and a biopsy before putting me on interferon treatments ASAP.

I received your book about this same time and placed my first order on January 24th. My iron-binding test came back with all the numbers in the acceptable range, but my ALT had risen to 65. On January 25, I added your therapy suggestions to what I was already taking. I asked for one more test before committing to a biopsy. That test was done on February 11th. The results were reported to me on February 18th. After adding your therapy, my viral load dropped to 333,350 and my ALT dropped to 52 in less than a month.

As of this writing, my specialist is still out of town and is unaware of the massive drop in viral activity that these numbers represent, but his nurse practitioner and my GP are very aware of the unprecedented results. In the hopes that my experience may well be of benefit to other patients, they were anxious to know exactly what I had done, and I have explained my treatment plan to them, including detailed information along with a copy of your book.

Much credit is due to you for your exhaustive efforts in seeking out and compiling the information in your books and making them available to those facing the challenge of hepatitis C. I must also give the ultimate credit to God. In Hosea 4:6 God says, "My people perish for a lack of knowledge." Then in Proverbs 2:6 he says, "For the Lord gives wisdom." Mainstream, conventional medicine lacks sufficient knowledge of this disease to offer a cure. God offers both wisdom and healing through His Son. I am thankful that God has entrusted you with a key element of His wisdom to bring hope and results to those confronted with the disease and the uncertain results of conventional treatment.

My next test is scheduled for March 11th. I look forward to seeing another dramatic drop: zero viral load with all other levels normal!

Sincerely,
Don, Minnesota

I've received over 50,000 letters and e-mails from those suffering with hepatitis C. My book entitled: *HEPATITIS C FREE, ALTERNATIVE MEDICINE VS. THE DRUG INDUSTRY: THE PEOPLE SPEAK* contains hundreds of them, a few of which are printed here:

Hi, Lloyd,

"I just wanted to tell you how much I appreciate you making your story available on the Internet. When my husband was diagnosed with hepatitis C, the first place I went was the net. I know that the AMA has only one objective; to keep their pockets filled while never "curing" anything. Although my uncle is head of Pathology at Penrose Hospital in Colorado Springs, and my husband's brother is a doctor in Chicago, I have learned that the best "drugs" for the human body are the natural ones. When my mom was diagnosed 5 years ago with PBC, I worked hard to get her to go to a naturopath, which she finally did and for the past 3 years her enzyme tests have been normal. She had a massive stroke in '75 and had been on so many drugs since then-no wonder her liver was compromised!

I read your book, and what a nightmare you went through. I am glad that you are well now. When the GI doctor talked to us last week he, of course, said interferon was the "only" treatment. I was armed with all the info from the Internet and asked him about natural herbal treatment, and this meek little man turned into a demon denouncing herbs and the fact that they are "not tested, regulated or pure" and that he wouldn't give "that stuff" to his own wife. I politely pointed out that all synthetic drugs pass through the liver and compromise it. He made a few more comments about the "efficacy" of interferon, so I shut my mouth, realizing he was another closed-minded AMA robot. He wrote in my husband's records: "wife does not approve of treatment." GOOD! I want them to be aware that I am not going to stand by and watch these VA butchers kill my husband.

Sorry this is long winded. I am so grateful for all your research and compassion toward others that are suffering from this disease. I am confident that the information you have provided along with a good naturopath doctor, that my husband will be cured. Again, a great big Thanks!"

Sincerely,
Marcia

Hi, Lloyd,

"I started to read your book. There are so many interesting things and this is a book from one patient to other patients. This makes all the difference. I was shocked when I was reading that your health insurance canceled your policy. In Europe we don't have the same system and you can always go to the hospital, even when you are without a job. Keep up the good work."

Bye,
Cinzia

Dear Lloyd,

"I have a lot of faith and I believe that it is not over for me. I have begun taking aloe vera, Liver Detox, and milk thistle because I nearly died from the interferon combination. I actually thought I was going to die before I got better and my doctor told me to keep on taking it. I couldn't even climb up the stairs because of weakness. My liver and my stomach swelled and I felt lousy. He told me that the herbs weren't proven when I told him my body wasn't agreeing with what he was saying. My stomach is still a little swollen but not as bad and I don't have any pain. I lead a natural active life and this diagnosis has been devastating, but your book has given me hope."

Sincerely,
Alice

Hi, Lloyd,

"I have hepatitis C and have been through all the conventional treatments of interferon. I initially had 6 months of injections of 3 million units 3 times per week. But my counts still weren't normal. My doctor referred me to the University of Florida Shands teaching hospital where Dr. Gary Davis was conducting a study for Shearing Plough. The study used the same treatment of 3 million units 3 times per week...when I still had high AST ALT levels; I was then given 5 million units 3 times week, until I developed such horrendous side effects that my doctor contacted Dr. Davis and had me removed from the study. When I stopped the study my AST was 128 and my ALT was 189. That was after several years of the interferon combination treatment. During the course of this extended treatment I got mouth sores, lost most of my hair, was constantly exhausted and sick to my stomach, and I became increasingly depressed. I also saw things that were not there but in my case I had never experienced depression in my life and I am in my 50's. I now live with depression. I had been told that interferon would leave your body once you stopped taking it. But in my case there seems to have been permanent damage to my brain pathways including the ones dealing with serotonin. It also affected my memory and I now have ADD. Since my liver is already in advanced cirrhosis I started taking milk thistle tablets as well as other parts of your program against my doctor's advice. My ALT is now 32 and my AST 35. Of course my doctor still isn't convinced and won't be until it's proven by medical science that your program, instead of a spontaneous remission, healed me."

Steve H.

To Lloyd:

"Wanted you to know that I have been on the program you suggested, plus a thymic formula from a Dr. Burgstiner in Georgia, for a few days short of 3 months. I got my first test results today and my ALT count has gone from 398 to 37 I want them to test for the virus but they haven't done that yet. Thanks for your help."

"I feel so great after getting some positive results that I want everyone to know. I went through the same thing you did with the combination therapy of interferon and ribavirin. It got so bad that I couldn't even brush my own hair. I still have trouble with my mood swings but I am more positive than I have been in a long time and I hope that will help. Thanks for your help."

From: LB

Dear Lloyd:

"If it wasn't for you I don't know where I would be. I could not think straight, I could not drive, and it was horrible. Now life is wonderful! One month on your program and I drove 8 hours to Maine and I didn't even get tired. Then I went to Colorado and went skiing for the first time in years. I can't thank you enough. After 60 days, my viral load has dropped from 663,260 to less than 100,780. You are such an inspiration to me and I pray for you every night."

Grace

Lloyd,

"Excellent book! It works well for individuals looking for the kind of help you offer. I am recommending it to all of my hepatitis patients."

Dr.

Lloyd,

"After reading your book, I began taking milk thistle and drinking teas. In two months my ALT dropped from 103 to 44. My AST also dropped from 130 to 76 and I haven't touched any interferon. Lloyd, your book has been the best inspiration for me. I'm sure I'll be talking to you again soon. I am impressed, you're **THE MAN!**"

G.N.

Dear Lloyd,

"I've seen my dear friend go from standing on death's door to being a vital and healthy man again. He did it by following a program that he has since written into his book, *Triumph Over Hepatitis C*. Having been in the rock and roll business in the crazy 70s, I witnessed a lot of abusive behavior by people I admired. Some of those people are no longer with us but many of them, like Eric Clapton (who's band I was in for 4 years), turned their lives around and totally cleaned up their acts. Without the help that's available to people who need it and ask for it, I doubt many of us would have succeeded. For alcoholics and drug addicts there is AA and NA, and various other support groups. For people with hepatitis C there is good proven advice in Lloyd Wright's book. If you know anyone who is suffering from this devastating health problem, before you even go near interferon, try everything else you can to help-including getting this book for them. As I have seen in my friend, it WORKS!"

Sincerely,

Yvonne Elliman

Dear Lloyd,

"I am writing to share my success and thank you for your work with the hepatitis C virus. I am 48 years old. Although I did some wild and crazy things in the 70's, for the past 20 years I have maintained a lifestyle of healthy living.

This summer I applied for a life insurance policy. Imagine my surprise and shock when I was denied coverage due to testing positive for hepatitis C.

I went to the web and read stories of doom and gloom from the medical community. Then I visited your site! I ordered your book immediately.

In the meantime, I went to my family doctor who blew this off as "no big deal." He said it was like being on a slow moving train on a long track, that I would probably live with it, rather than die from it. He said I should probably have a follow up in about a year and gave me the name of a gastroenterologist.

Your book came and I read it the first night. I ordered the supplements right away, tried to follow your regime as closely as possible, including the NatCell thymus, which as you know is very expensive.

I went to the gastroenterologist and he wanted me to start interferon. I said, "No, it's not really known to work." He agreed. He wanted to schedule me for a liver biopsy. I said, "No, its not really going to alter my course." He said, "Start taking milk thistle, it's the only known thing to work. He didn't say how much to take or where to get it. That was O.K. I already knew.

I had been on the supplements for about a week when I went to my chiropractor. He said to me, "I don't know what it is, but you're putting your body through some tremendous changes." That's when I told him about the HCV and starting the homeopathic supplements. He altered

236

his technique that day to work on the area of the spine that controls the liver function.

I am happy to report that after only 5 weeks of your therapy in combination with my chiropractor, my SGOT (AST) has decreased from 86 to 38 (a reduction of 56% and in some lab reference ranges considered to be within the normal). My SGPT (ALT) has decreased from 112 to 54 (a reduction of almost 52%). Viral load was not drawn on the first set of labs so I have no baseline, but on the second lab draw my viral load was 8,000.

I recently added milk thistle and mushroom teas to my regime. I plan to have my labs drawn every three months, the next one around mid-November. I will let you know the results, but again expect to beat this. Again, thank you for sharing your work."

Bob

Hi, Lloyd,

"Just wanted to share the news. I have cleared the virus. Thanks for all of your kindness and support.

Lisa R.

Hi, Lloyd!

"I really can't express how much your program means to me—I mean it's my LIFE! I am a 39 year old female, I found out I had this last summer and was obsessed with the seemingly endless ramifications—it felt like my life was truly over. I took some of the supplements, but started on almost all of the program in Feb. 2001 (all except cat's claw and hyssop teas and I dropped hepastat in March, so really all of it.) Like most, I had horrible experiences with a gastroenterologist who really pushed for a biopsy and touted the great benefits of pegylated interferon, which would "knock the virus out of me." I knew, from you, that

237

the only thing that would be knocked out was me, so I went for the ultrasound which said no damage found and refused the biopsy—there was no reason for it, and that would definitely cause scarring to the liver. Your site has given me endless hope, especially lately as more great test results come in. Now for mine. On 12/22/00, ALT = 76, AST = 52, PCR Quant = 89,336 copies/ml (and IU/ml = 31,700 the other way to measure it?). On 8/10/01, ALT = 16, AST = 19, PCR Quant = 1,558 (under 1,000 is non-detected) (and IU/ml = 649, under 600 is non-detected). My gastro. received these results, knows I'm taking "supplements" and hasn't even contacted me to see what I'm doing to get such great results—I guess if he doesn't have a cure, no one can. From others' experiences, do you have any idea how long it takes to get to zero (zero!) from here? Anyway, to everyone out there—keep plugging—IT WORKS! If insurance would pay for this program, think of how much it would save them in the long run. I'm faxing the labs to you, and am just THRILLED about the results! Thanks again."

S.

Hi, Lloyd—

"I want to let you know I have a friend, Joel, who had Hep C and he went on Natcell and all the herbs and basically he told me he just went on a GODZILLA TYPE … remedy. He took Natcell, frozen Thymus, and the frozen liver for about a month along with Transfactor. He went to his doctor and had extensive blood work done and the doctor said he no longer has Hep C. They could not find a trace.

Lloyd, this guy couldn't even get out of bed in the morning. He doesn't have a computer so I am delivering the message. I am going to go have my blood work done soon after the holidays and see how far I have come along. I know one thing is for sure, I do feel a whole lot better and I am expecting to hear better news about my condition with Hep C. Thanx a Million and God bless you, Lloyd."

Mark R.

February 16, 2002

This 52-year-old male called me yesterday and faxed me his blood work because his doctor did not have time to explain it. He was on my program for two months when his doctor convinced him to try peg intron for a study being offered.

When he stopped my program his viral load was 1.904.149. That was 11/29/00. Six months of peg intron and his viral load was 4.455.710.

He told me a good day on peg intron was a day he could 'lift his head off the pillow!' That is an exact quote.

He started back on my program, realizing he had to live with this and interferons are not life friendly.

On 9/18/01 his viral load was 3.570.492.

His next test was on 1/9/02. His viral load was 2.160.289. His SGOT 32, his SGPT 35, Protein, total, serum 7.2 Bilirubin total 0.5.

The rest of his blood work is also perfect with the exception of WBC count; RBC count and Platelet count being on the low side as a direct result of the negative side effects of peg intron. Blood tests on file.

Lloyd

March 14, 2002

A local client and noted successful Malibuite recently purchased *Triumph Over Hepatitis C* at the local health food store. He came and visited me two months ago.

His viral load was 480.090, blood drawn on 11/06/01. He started my program in full in mid-January. On Feb. 28,

2002, his HCV RNA Quantitative viral load IU/ml is 99.419. **This represents over an 80% drop in two months.**

Dr. Sammy Saab at UCLA did not seem impressed. The client is extremely happy that he is getting well without being disabled by peg intron.

Blood tests on file!

Lloyd

Greetings:

On March 19, 2002 at 10:13 a.m., D.B., a female client of mine, called me and said she has been on my program for eight weeks. She contracted the HCV 15 years ago during the birth of her daughter. She is, or I should say 'was' geno type 1A.

At eight weeks she tested non-detected for the hepatitis C virus. Both of her doctors, a gynecologist and a pediatrician, could not believe it so they tested her again.

In contrast to so many of the closed-minded doctors I hear about, both of these doctors wanted to know what she did instead of saying it was a spontaneous remission, which is what I hear a lot from doctors when one becomes non-detected from use of my program. They both called me with great interest.

Congratulations to D.B. in New Jersey and to her interested doctors. The Dragon can be slain by doing what is in *Triumph Over Hepatitis C.*

Lloyd

Good Morning!

"Just wanted to update you on my progress. Started your program on my birthday, February 20, 2002, about 45 days ago. My urine is back to normal, no more gray, inching is gone, brain fog is gone for most part, have more energy working 12 hours a day, 5 to 5.

240

I did pick up my one year old's cold after being up with him 72 hours straight last weekend; however, within 5 days was able to beat it (prior was 2 to 3 weeks with cold). Very excited about future with my wife and kids!

Just wanted to thank you once again."

J.F.

Dear Lloyd,

"I was diagnosed with Hep C in December 2000. At that time my alt was 148. In Jan. 2001 I began your program. In March, 2001 I had another blood test and my alt was 61. HCV RNA PCR Quant 191,000. In April, 2001 I took another test prior to gallbladder surgery, alt was 46, IICV RNA PCR Quant 137,000.

I was thrilled but my doctor said it didn't mean anything as I wasn't taking anything he recognized as a cure and the liver enzymes were still high. I continued on your program but not as aggressively as I should, as this ass of a doctor? put so many doubts in me. I felt better but thought it was because there was no more gallbladder pain or problems.

For the hell of it I took another test last week (after a lot of stress and wine) and today got the results. Are you ready for this??? Alt 34-normal and HCV RNA PCR Quant 2590 !!!!!

I will get aggressive from now on as I want to prove there is a cure. Next year this time, if not before, my blood will be free of this virus.

Thank you for—whatever—just THANK YOU!!"

Ron

Lloyd,

"Hope all is well with you! Today is 4 weeks on the program. (I mean "ON" the Program!) I have not missed one herb or tea. I even modify my schedule to accommodate making the teas, etc. This is quite time-consuming, as you know. I do feel better, and I am cautiously optimistic. I absolutely cannot afford this; however, I have decided I would rather live in the poorhouse than die with the help of the doctor's free Peg and Ribo. I will tell you that my body is sending me signs that this is working ...

Sounds weird, but all of those people who are doing what I am certainly understand, as do you.

For the last two and a half years my doctors have been trying to figure out my dizziness... two CAT scans and 4 MRIs, two neurologists, etc. ... in the last two weeks my dizziness is gone.

For about one year I feel like I was old, tired, fatigues, laid on the couch all the time ... I am back to working with energy, golfing, fishing, yard work, I feel like I used to.

After 2 or 3 years of shoulder and knee pain that the doctors said could only be fixed with surgery, my knees don't hurt at all, my right shoulder hurts once in a while. Both shoulders used to hurt 24 hours a day.

The "baseball" under my ribs is 98% gone. When I wake up in the morning, I am awake when I open my eyes. It used to take me an hour to 'get going.'

This is after 30 days of your natural program. It's no wonder the drug companies don't want people to know, but so very, very sad.

Just like all the others, Lloyd... I want to thank you. You and what you are doing is an answer to prayer. Without this answer, I would not have found you at all. I can only imagine. My prayers will continue for you and yours.

D.S.

Lloyd,

"I just received my recent liver panel and viral load tests. I'm jazzed. My history is as follows:

I was diagnosed with Hep C in 1997. My AST was 49 and my ALT was 60 and my viral load was >1,000,000. Over the years my numbers stayed the same or lower.

I read your book and went on the full program in 10/01. My base test in 9/01 before I started the program were a little disturbing: AST 98, ALT 109 and viral load was >1,000,000.

Here's my progression since being on the program with specific viral load numbers.

12/1/01
AST 65, ALT 23, GGT 28
RNA, QN, PCR – 5,560,000 copies/ml
RNA PCR – 2,440,000 IU/ml
2/1/02
AST 54, ALT 29, GGT 29
RNA, QN, PCR – 4,280,000 copies/ml
RNA PCR – 1,720,000 IU/ml
5/1/02
AST 45, ALT 24, GGT 28
RNA, QN, PCR – 1,610,000 copies/ml
RNA PCR – 596,000 IU/ml

As you can see, my recent liver panel is in the normal range except my AST and my viral load has come down consistently and significantly. I'm on the program 100% including teas, frozen thymus and herbal supplements. I also eat extremely well and I work out around two hours per day. I feel really good! I think I am on the home stretch of becoming Hep C free. Also, your web page is excellent along with the quality of your herbs and products. Your company gets an A+ for timely and accurate order deliveries. Please feel free to print this great journey.

Sincerely, and Thanks, J.

Lloyd,

After 17 months of interferon-ribavirin and 3 months of pegylated interferon with some response of the hep c virus (non lasting), my viral load went right back up after I discontinued use - not to mention the devastating side effects to myself.

I finally ended up with a doctor who was at USC for the first interferon trials where they discovered that raising the dosage just ended up putting patients in the hospital with no real gain. He looked at me and told me I had had enough interferon and that, by the way, it takes six months for the devastating side effects to wear off.

Approximately 11 months ago I started on your frozen thymus and the vitamins etc., as spelled out in your book. My viral load is down to 183,000 as of a month ago, no side effects. Also my fevers and flu-like systems have tapered off, once again with NO SIDE EFFECTS.

Thanks again for doing all the research and pioneering a path out of this hepatitis c nightmare.

G.A.

Dear Lloyd & Staff:

Just wanting to wish you a Merry Christmas and Happy New Year! By the grace of God and your products we are now Hepatitis C Free! Enclosed are some copies of our blood work.

Our doctor was very impressed as we are his only patients to beat this with your products. We gave our doctor a copy of your book and he is going to refer some of his patients to us to help tell about this method of healing. Thank God we will never take interferon again as it was the worse drug with side effects we have ever taken.

Thanking you again for all your help!

The above is a type written copy of a hand written letter I received in early December 2003.

Enclosed in the envelope are 4 blood tests.

2 for B.L.:

One dated 12/30/2002 stating, Hep C detected

One dated 12/04/2003 stating, Hep C not detected

2 for her husband, H.L.:

One dated 12/30/2002 stating, Hep C detected

One dated 12/30/2003 stating, Hep C not detected

I spoke with these people on the phone a few times. They had tried interferon years earlier and described it as "JUST HELL, ROCKED MY WORLD!" It did not work; viral load went up 3 times higher than when they started.

They also said that the doctors treated them like second-class citizens.

The doctors did not give them any hope as interferon had failed.

They both give credit to God and this was the best Christmas present they could have.

Both of these people did most of my full program from April 2003 to December 2003.

They were both geno-type 2A.

I have their blood tests on file.

Lloyd

BLOOD TESTS RELATING TO HEPATITIS C.
HEPATITIS C GENOTYPES

Isolates of hepatitis C virus are grouped into six major genotypes. These genotypes are sub-typed according to sequence characteristics and are designated as 1a, 1b, 1c, 2a, 2b, 2c, 3a, 3b, 4a-h and 6a.

LIVER FUNCTION TESTS:

AST (SGOT)
Increase of aspartate aminotransferase (AST, formerly called SGOT) is seen in any condition involving necrosis of hepatocytes, myocardial cells, or skeletal muscle cells.
Put simply, this is a liver function test that measures liver enzymes and inflammation.

ALT (SGPT)

Increase of serum alanine aminotransferase (ALT, formerly called SGPT) is seen in any condition involving necrosis of hepatocytes, myocardial cells, erythrocytes, or skeletal muscle cells.

Again, this is a liver function test that measure liver enzymes and inflammation.

BILIRUBIN

Serum total bilirubin is increased in hepatocellular damage (infectious hepatitis, alcoholic, and other toxic hepatopathy, neoplasmas), intra- and extra-hepatic biliary tract obstruction.

ALBUMIN

Decreased serum albumin is seen in states of decreased synthesis (malnutrition, malabsorption, liver disease, and other chronic diseases.)

PCR – POLYMERASE CHAIN REACTION

This test is used to measure the viral load of the hepatitis C virus in the RNA. Hepatitis C is an RNA virus unlike most other viruses, which are DNA viruses.

This test is currently performed in many different ways and results are often confusing and especially frustrating. Most tests are range tests indicating whether the viral load is greater than 850.000 or greater than 1,000,000. These are range tests.

Most doctors tell patients, "If it's over 850.000, it's bad." This is not true. The viral load of a specific person is not related to ALT and AST levels, symptoms, or liver damage.

When requesting a PCR, ask for "PCR HCV RNA QUANTITATIVE (VIRAL LOAD)—specific number.

(New tests are constantly emerging. See message board at www.HepatitisCFree.com for updates).

THE HEPATITIS A AND/OR B VACCINE <u>WILL</u> RAISE YOUR VIRAL LOAD.

There is still very little information "out there" about what may negatively affect the viral load. But I have years of experience speaking with people infected with HCV, reviewing their lab results and drawing correlations between their viral loads and related events. And I can tell you that vaccines, certain pharmaceuticals and even medical and dental procedures do negatively affect viral load. The correlation between vaccines and an increased viral load is so strong, in fact, that I feel I should warn you: Your Hepatitis C viral load will most likely triple and may even go up by tens of millions if you get the Hepatitis A and B vaccines, the flu vaccine or any vaccine that puts a load on the immune system. Please note: I am not advising you against getting such vaccinations, just warning you of what usually happens.

IRON BINDING TEST

This is a very important test, which is often overlooked by doctors. You will not improve until your iron levels are in the normal range. Iron overload usually occurs in men, but I have encountered it in women as well; about 25% of men, 8% of pre-menopausal women and 30% of post-menopausal women who have hepatitis C also have iron overload. Phlebotomy used to be the quickest, cheapest method to lower iron levels. Now there is a product called IP-6 (inositol hexaphosphate) that is as effective as phlebotomy. Within 1-3 months of normalizing your ferritin (see below) level, your ALT and AST should follow.

FERRITIN TEST

Ferritin is a complex of iron and protein mainly found in the liver that is one of the forms in which iron is stored in the body. So in that sense, a ferritin test is more specific than an iron test to the liver and to hepatitis C. But please try to get both tests, as they should both be normal in order for your health to improve.

ALPHA FETA PROTEIN (ALF) is produced by people with hepatic carcinoma or germ cell tumors. Approximately 79-90% of people with Hepatacellular carcinoma will have levels that range from above normal 20 ng/ml to 10,000,000 ng/ml. A small elevation in ALP may occur in people with non-malignant disease such as cirrhosis or viral hepatitis. This test should be accompanied with an ultra sound to confirm results.

PLATELET COUNT – Measures the number of platelets and reflects your ability to clot blood.

IN CLOSING

Unfortunately, over the past forty years, the prevailing health care system and the government agencies entrusted to regulate them have virtually excluded treatments related to so-called alternative, traditional, or unorthodox medicine. Especially kept in competitive check have been herbs and other nutritional supplements, which hundreds of studies have demonstrated possess the potential to replace many modern synthesized pharmaceutical drugs. A repression of health-care alternatives has been achieved both directly through regulatory control and indirectly through what would appear to be a systematic offensive against alternative health care providers.

The government has required that any time a health claim about an herb or dietary supplement is made, the producers must prove that the supplement is a safe and effective drug. While this seems fair enough, the reality is that a new drug application costs up to $359 million, take eight years or more to process and, most ironically, can never actually result in a patent because a whole herb is a substance that cannot be patented. It is somewhat of a foreign concept in the era of modern medicine's magic bullets to imagine that nutrition, herbs, and supplements benefit so many parts of the human body.

Alternative medicine means that there is another option in medicinal treatment, particularly when the ones we are accustomed to relying on prove ineffective. While I may seem at times in opposition to modern medicine, the reality is that I have been forced to be, simply by taking the position of being open to the credible healing benefits of herbs and nutritional supplements. In actuality, I hope that both conventional and alternative medicine can unite and thus expand, enabling people to choose their treatment of choice while being supported by their insurance companies and doctors.

In the case of hepatitis C, it is a proven fact that what the medical community is offering as treatment at this time still does not work and in fact exacerbates the condition. In my own case of hepatitis C, I turned first to conventional medicine for healing. When interferon failed to work, and in actual fact made me more ill, I had no choice but to explore and self-prescribe a treatment of natural remedies that ultimately became my cure. Having shared my therapy with thousands of hepatitis C victims, I now know with certainty that what worked for me also works for others. It is therefore my opinion, based on the results reported to me, that this program works better than anything currently offered by the FDA. To view hundreds of testimonials, read *Hepatitis C Free, Alternative Medicine vs. The Drug*

Industry, The People Speak. If you have any hesitation regarding anything in this book, you can find confirmation there written by countless others in their own words.

A good solid belief in God, a structured life, and self-awareness are necessary to achieve success in anything. If you are not disciplined, begin learning.

REFERENCES

1. Informational and Solicitation Letter from the American Liver Foundation, 1998.
2. Marohn, Stephanie "Naomi Judd, For the Country Queen, Alternative Medicine Rules" *Alternative Medicine Digest*, Issue 21, January 1998, pages 68-72.
3. *Hepatology, A Texbook of Liver Disease*, David Zakim, M.D. and Thomas D. Boyer, M.D., 2nd Ed., Vol. 2, pp. 980-81
4. "Placebos and Positive Belief Help Healing," *Hepatitis Alert*, Hepatitis Foundation International, Fall 1998, page 5.
5. U.S. News on CNN Internet, August 23, 1997, page 3.
6. Los Angeles Times, Part B Metro, February 23, 1994, page 3.
7. Satchell, Michael and Hedges, Stephen *U.S. News and World Report Online*, Sept 1, 1997, page 3.
8. Hall, Carl T. "Scientist Stalk a Quiet Killer, Sci Clone, Chiron Seek Hepatitis C Treatment," *San Francisco Chronicle*, July 21, 1995.
9. Phone conversation with Pat Conely 6/11/99. For further information contact: Price-Pottenger Nutrition Foundation, P.O. Box 2614 La Mesa, CA 91943-2614, 619-574-7763 or www.PRICE-Pottenger-org.
10. Rohrer, Jean "Healing Light: Milk Thistle," Internet, Pages 1-3.
11. N. Kouttab et al., "Thymomodulin: Biological Properties and Clinical Applications." *Med. Oncol. And Tumor Pharmacother*. Vol. 6, pp. 5-9, 1989.
12. W. Hemmings, "Dietary Protein Reaches the Brain." *Orthomol. Psychiatry*, Vol. 6, pp. 309-16, 1977.
13. C. Ziovdrou et al. "Opiod Peptides Derived from Food Proteins." *J. Biol. Chem.*, Vol. 254, pp. 2446-49, 1979.
14. R. Bradford & H. Allen. *Oxidology*. Chula Vista, CA: R.W. Bradford Foundation, 1997.
15. Whitaker, Julian "Longevity Science Biopro Thymic Protein A," *Health and Healing*, March 1997.

16. Radchenko VG, et al., "The efficacy of immunomodulating preparations in treating patients with chronic cholestatic liver disease," *Vrachebnoe Delo.* 1992 Nov-Dec, (11-12): 38.

17. Berkow R., et al., *The Merck Manual of Diagnosis*, Merck Research Laboratories, Rathway, NJ. 1992, p. 308.

18. *Hepatology*, April 2000, pp. 1022-1024, Vol. 31, No 4.

19. Yale Article (editorial), "Do Natural T Cells Promote Liver Regeneration. *Hepatology*, April 2000, pp. 1022-1024, Vol. 31, No. 4.

20. Fausto, N., et al., "Liver regeneration. Role of growth factors and cytokines in hepatic regeneration," *Journal of FASEB*, Vol. 9, No. 15, pp. 1527-1536, Dec. 1999

21. Teir, H. and Ravanti, K Experimental Cell Research. Vol. 5, p. 500, 1953.

22. Blomqvist, K. "Acta Path,". *Microbiol. Scaand, Suppl.* Vol. 121, 1957.

23. Levi, J.U. and Zeppa, R.J. *Surgical Research.* Vol. 12, p. 114, 1972.

24. Compagno, J. and Grisham, *J. Western Federal Proceedings*, Vol. 32, p. 837, 1973.

25. Lloyd, E.A., et al., *British Journal of Experimental Pathology*, Vol. 55, p. 251, 1974.

26. Starzl, T.E., et al., "Growth-stimulating factor in regenerating canine liver." *The Lancet.*, January 20, 1979, pp. 127-130.

27. Michalopoulos, G.K. *Journal of FASEB*, Vol. 4, pp. 176-187, 1990.

28. Russell, W.E. and DuBois, R.N., *Liver Disease in Children*, (Suchy, F.J. and Craven, L., Eds.) (St. Louis: Mosby, 1994), pp. 11-30.

29. LaBrecque, D. *American Journal of Gastroenterology.* 69:S86S96, 1994.

30. Sporn, M.B. and Roberts, A.B., "Peptide growth factors and inflammation, tissue repair and cancer." *Journal of Clinical Investigation*, Vol. 78, pp. 329-332, 1986.

31. Sporn, M.B. and Roberts, A.B. "Peptide growth factors are multifunctional." *Nature,* Vol. 332, pp.217-219.

32. Barkai, A. and McQuaid, C. "Predator-prey role reversal in a marine benthic ecosystem." *Science,,* Vol. 242, pp. 62-64, 1988.

33. Sehgal, P.B., et al., "Human Beta-2 interferon and B-cell differentiation factor BSF-2 are identical." *Science.*, Vol 235, pp. 731-732, 1987.

34. Kishimoto, T. and Hirano, T. "Molecular regulation of 6-lymphocyte response," *Annual Review of Immunology*, Vol. 6, pp. 485-512, 1988.

35. Nimer, S.D., et al., "Serum cholesterol lowering activity of granulocyte-macrophage colony-stimulating factor." *Journal of the American Medical Association*, Vol. 260, pp. 3297-3300, 1988.

36. Saito, H., et al., "Enhancing effect of the liver extract and flavin adenine Dinucleotide mixture on anti-viral efficacy of interferon in patients with chronic hepatitis C." *Keio Journal of Medicine.*, Vol. 45, No. l, pp. 48-53, March 1996.

37. Ibid

38. Nelson, C, et al., "Giycerophosphoryiethanolamine (GPEA) identified as an hepatocyte growth stimulator in liver extracts." *Experimental Cell Research*, Vol. 229, No. l, pp. 20-26, Nov. 1996.

39. Akatsu, T., et al., "On the activities of parathyroid hormone-like factor and transforming growth factors in extract of pancreatic cancer associated with humoral hypercalcemia of malignancy." *Acta Endocrinology* (Copenhagen), Vol. 118, No. 2, pp. 232-238, June 1988.

40. Ueno, N., et al., "Purification and partial characterization of mitogenic factor from bovine liver: structural homology with basic fibroblast growth factor." *Regulation Pept.*, Vol. 16, No. 2, pp. 135-145, Dec. 1986.

41. Rodriguez-Fragoso, L. "Physiologic and physiopathologic role of hepatocyte growth factor." *Review of Investigational Clinics*, Vol. 50, No. 4, pp. 355-367, July/Aug. 1998.

42. Balkovetz, D.F. and Lipschutz, J.H. "Hepatocyte growth factor and the kidney: it is not just for the liver."

International Review of Cytology, Vol. 186, pp. 225260, 1999.

43. Matsumoto, K. and Nakamura, T. "HGF: its organotrophic role and therapeutic potential." *Ciba Foundation Symposium*, Vol. 212, pp. 198-211, 1997.

44. Michalopoulos, G.K. and DeFrances, M.C. "Liver regeneration." *Science,* Vol. 276, (5309): 60-66, Apr. 4 1997.

45. Morton Walker, M.D.

46. Law, David, "Medical Mushrooms: An Ancient Alternative to Synthetic Drugs, A Positive Approach to Health and Wellness," Internet, pages 1-3

47. Packer, Ester, *Alpha-Lipoic Acid: The Universal Antioxidants,* pp.2-3, 1997

48. Mowrey, Dan, "Licorice for the Female Reproductive System," H*ealth Store News*, June/July, 1995.

49. Lust, John, *The Herb Book*, Bantam Books, New York, 1974.

50. David, Brent W., *A New World Class Herb for A. K. Practice*, 1992

51. Finnegan, Dr. John, *The Healing Aloe: Nature's Wondrous Gift and Cancer Prevention and Recover: A Nutritional Approach*

52. Pitman, John C., *Immune Enhancing Effects of Aloe*

53. Heyman, Dr. Jeri L., *The Secret Promise of Aloe Vera,* Herbal Answers, Inc.

54. Larsen, Hans R., "Vitamin C: Your Ultimate Health Insurance," *International Health News.*

55. Carper, Jean, Vitamin C chapter in *The Food Pharmacy,* Bantam Books, New York, p. 222, 1999

56. Hanbury, Daniel, *Pharmaceutical Journal*, 1854

57. Morton Walker, D.P.M., *Townsend Letter for Doctors and Patients,* July 1996

58. James R. Privitera, M.D.

59. McMillan, S.I., *None of These Diseases*, Fleming H. Rand Co., 1984

60. *The Tony Brown Journal, The T.V. Series*, Show No. 1615, *The Life Factor,* 1996

61. *Blackwoods Materia Medic*, Economic Homeo Pharmacy, 1959

62. Williams, S. R., *Nutrition and Diet Therapy*, C.W. Mosby Co., 1969

63. Nutrition Search, Inc., *Nutrition Almanac,* McGraw Hill, 1975

64. Heinz International Research Center, *Heinz Nutritional Data,* 1972

65. Colimore, B., et al., *Nutrition and Your Body,* Light Wave, 1974

66. Clark, Linda, *Handbook of Natural Remedies for Common Ailments*, Devia Adair, 1976

67. Boericke, William, *Pocket Manual of Homeopathic Materia Medica*, Boericke & Runyon, 1972

68. Garrison, R.H., et al., *The Nutrition Desk Reference,* Keats Publishing, New Canaan, CT, 1985

69. Carper, Jean, *The Food Pharmacy,* pp. 105, 121, and 279, Bantam Books, New York, 1988

70. Shahani and Fernandes, "Anticarcinogenic and immuno-logical properties of dietary lactobacilli," *Journal of Food Protection,* Vol. 53, pp. 704-11

71. Oster, Kurt, "Milk: The Homogenization Deception," Internet, 1999

72. Aspartame/NutraSweet News Release, October 17, 1996, Aspartame (NutraSweet) Toxicity Information Center

73. Bazell, Robert, "Medical errors a major killer," NBC NEWS, November 19, 1999

74. Finnegan, Dr. John, "The Shocking Truth About Refined Oils," *Health Naturally,* August/September 1994, p. 20

Appendix A

Informational Article about Interferon alpha –2b
recombinant

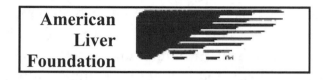

American Liver Foundation

INFORMATION
The Liver in Health and Disease

HEPATITIS C: THERAPY
Gary L. Davis, MD
University of Florida
Gainesville, Florida

Key Points:

1. Chronic hepatitis C is a heterogeneous disease whose natural history and response to treatment is probably influenced by multiple factors including but not limited to viral genotype, level of viral replication, and histology.

2. Interferon is the only agent of proven efficacy in the treatment of Hepatitis C. Standard treatment is Interferon alfa-2b at a dose of three million units three times a week. The initial course of treatment is 6 months, but <u>nearly all patients relapse and require re-treatment. The goal of Interferon treatment is suppression of active disease; this usually requires long-term therapy. Eradication of virus does not appear to be a realistic goal in most patients.</u>

3. Higher doses and longer duration of initial therapy have limited benefit over standard therapy. However,

higher initial doses may increase the interval before relapse and escalation of the dose may achieve response in some non-responders.

4. Treatment trials have tended to study relatively homogenous patient groups and the possibility of extrapolating these results to different patient populations is extremely limited. This is especially true of studies from geographic areas. Thus, future studies should: (1) consider genotype, viral load, and histology in stratification; and (2) include a control group of standard treatment for comparison.

5. Selection of patients for this chronic treatment remains controversial. Treatment of patients with active disease is most cost- effective, but other factors such as the degree of symptoms must be considered.

6. The definition of response to treatment is evolving as a technology of measurement of HCV improves. It is likely that future treatment strategies will be dependent upon virologic endpoints in addition to, or instead of, serum ALT.

7. Different agents and adjuncts have been incompletely studied to date. Ribavirin reduces serum ALT levels to normal and improves fatigue in nearly half of patients. Histology and virus levels do not appear to be significantly altered. The mechanism of its action of this interesting agent is not clear.

INTRODUCTION

The first trial of interferon as therapy for chronic non-A, non-B hepatitis was reported in 1986. This pilot study demonstrated that alpha Interferon therapy: (1) was effective at low doses (in comparison to doses previously shown to be required for hepatitis B and D); (2) decreased serum ALT levels promptly upon initiation of therapy, a pattern suggestive of an antiviral effect of Interferon; and (3) was usually associated with relapse when treatment was stopped, indicating a failure to eradicate the virus. Many subsequent controlled studies have now confirmed all of these original observations. A dose of 3 million units of recombinant Interferon alfa-2b thrice weekly for 6 months is the currently approved standard for initial therapy in the United States. With the discovery of the hepatitis C virus responsible for non-A, non-B hepatitis and the availability of moderately sensitive techniques for detaching the virus, it is now apparent that the biochemical response to Interferon (normalization of ALT) is associated with loss of detectable viremia; thus, the primary response of Interferon is indeed due to the antiviral effects of the drug. However, the high relapse rate confirms the earlier suspicion that interferon is usually unable to eradicate the virus, which persists at levels below the current limits of detection in serum, liver, or peripheral blood mononuclear cells.

It is apparent that the usual effect of Interferon in patients with chronic Hepatitis C who respond to this therapy is one of viral suppression, not eradication or cure. Sustained or prolonged response to treatment (persistently normal ALT levels) occurs in only 15-20% of patients and is often associated with detectable viremia despite the biochemical absence of apparent hepatic injury. The observations from these early studies are important and must be considered in establishing appropriate justification and goals for Interferon therapy in clinical practice. Several crucial points must be made:

1. Interferon therapy appears to eradicate or cure infection in only a small proportion of patients. Thus, cure is an unrealistic goal of current Interferon regimens.

2. Interferon is suppressive to the Hepatitis C virus. The goal of therapy should be to suppress infection to a degree that liver disease is minimized.

3. The currently approved regimen of therapy (3 million units 3x per week for 6 months) is sub-optimal. It should be considered as initial therapy, not as definitive therapy. The goal of chronic viral suppression will require prolonged therapy, re-treatment of relapse, or maintenance regimens

Currently, clinical and basic research in Hepatitis C is just beginning to shed light on the issues important to therapeutics in this confusing disease. It is now apparent that the disease course is only slowly progressive in most patients; thus, histology may be important in assessing the timing of therapeutic investigation. It is evident that the natural history is different between genotypes. The initial and long-term response to therapy is also affected by both genotype and the level of viremia.

The differences in response to Interferon therapy, which occur as a result of viral differences, are critical to clinical research in therapeutics. Literally dozens of studies of various interferon dose regimens have appeared to demonstrate superiority of every conceivable permutation of dosing to the currently accepted regimens. However, few have compared these novel and potentially useful regimens to standard dosing. Since genotypes are geographically diverse and have significant influence on response to interferon, trials conducted on one continent or even in different countries of regions within a continent are not comparable. Changes in therapeutic regimens from the current standard must be based on careful comparisons of different regimens among genotypically similar patients with similar viral loads. It is likely that a single dosing strategy is not appropriate for all patients. Differences in the Hepatitis C virus from country to country may warrant local modifications in interferon dosing. Unfortunately, this implies that the considerable effort and expense of clinical trials may have little applicability outside of the area where they are conducted. At a bare minimum, genotype and the degree of viremia need to be considered as stratification levels in designing future clinical trials.

Finally, the traditional marker for assessing treatment response is normalization of the serum ALT level. Although this endpoint was established before identification of the Hepatitis C virus, it appears to be as appropriate as measuring HCV-RNA for determining the initial response to Interferon, i.e. normalization of ALT is usually associated with loss of detectable virus from the serum. However, after discontinuation of Interferon, HCV-RNA usually becomes detectable well before re-evaluation of ALT (the traditional definition of relapse) occurs. In fact, viremia may be present for months to years after Interferon is stopped despite persistently normal ALT levels ("sustained remission"). Other markers include aGST, procollagen III, and chocolate clearance, are under study and may serve as adjunctive markers of response. Clearly, future studies should consider alternative markers of response and relapse, which might prove to be more clinically useful than those currently employed.

TREATMENT OF CHRONIC HEPATITIS C

Standard Therapy

Standard initial therapy for chronic Hepatitis C infection is recombinant Interferon alfa-2b at a dose of 3 x 106 units administered subcutaneously 3 times per week for

263

6 months. This regimen is based on the results of 3 randomized controlled trials, which employed an identical protocol and were conducted in France and the United States. These trials demonstrated that 41% of patients normalized the serum ALT level during treatment and 70% of responders had histological improvement. Response to treatment is greatest in those patients without advanced inflammation or cirrhosis, high HCV-RNA levels, of genotypes 1a and 1b (Simmonds). Almost all responders (normal ALT) lose detectable HCV-RNA by reverse transcription polymerase chain reaction (RT-PCR) by the end of therapy. However, relapse occurs in 50-70% of patients after the end of the initial course and is associated with return of detectable HCV-RNA. Relapse usually responds to re-treatment with Interferon.

Alternative regimens: Higher dose, Longer duration.

The best way to improve the efficacy of interferon treatment is to improve the initial response and its durability. Controlled trials of alternative regimens including higher doses, daily dosing or longer durations of therapy have not shown that these schedules improve the response rate. However, higher doses of Interferon may increase the durability of the initial response, i.e. reduce early relapse. The effect of tapering the dose after the initial 6 months on subsequent relapse is unclear, having been reported to either reduce or have no effect on relapse. These findings need to be confirmed.

Adjuncts to Interferon Therapy
& Combination Therapy

Several compounds have been suggested to improve the response to Interferon in patients with chronic hepatitis C.

Ursodeoxycholic acid has been proposed as either a single agent or adjunct to Interferon, but its effects on viral replication and inflammation have been incompletely examined. NSAIDS have a potential role in augmenting the antiviral effects of Interferon through their ability to block prostaglandin synthesis, increase the epoxygenase pathway, and increase 2', 5' oligoadenylate synthetase, one of the effectors of Interferon activity. These effects have not been proven in vivo. N-acetyl cysteine (NAC), an antioxidant and glutathione source, has been shown in one pilot study to induce response to interferon when patients had previously failed to respond. However, most patients with chronic Hepatitis C are not glutathione deficient and the therapy is expensive and distasteful. Controlled trials need to determine if NAC has any effects in chronic Hepatitis C.

Ribavirin has not proven to significantly increase response to interferon in a single published study. However, several pilots studies published in abstract form suggest a possible effect. This agent's role has only begun to be explored. No scientific rationale exists for prednisone pretreatment in chronic Hepatitis C. Corticosteroids increase HCV replication. Nonetheless, prednisone pre-treatment has been shown in one study in the Orient to increase the durability of response. These findings need to be reexamined in a controlled fashion in genotyped patients.

Alternatives to Interferon

There are few alternatives to interferon on the horizon for patients with HCV infection. Thymosin is not effective. Ribavirin shows some promise as a single agent in the treatment of chronic Hepatitis C, but its effects are difficult to interpret. Although ribavirin is a nucleoside analogue and know antiviral agent, its ability to normalize serum ALT levels and improve symptoms in patients with chronic HCV infection does not appear to result from inhibition of HCV (viral levels remain unchanged). It is possible that the agent acts through inhibition of some effectors of tissue damage. Certainly, clarification of the mechanism of action of this agent will help define the pathogenesis of hepatic injury in HCV infection.

PROBLEMS WITH TREATMENT OF CHRONIC HEPATITIS C:

Interferon therapy of chronic HCV infection is not straight-forward. Therapy is initially effective in only a portion of patients and it appears that eradication of infection is unusual in patient infected with the genotypes most common in the United States and most areas of Europe. Thus, several issues are important in understanding the appropriateness and limitations of Interferon treatment.

Selection of Patients

Treatment of patients should be directed at those who will benefit from the intervention. Several issues are important to defining this benefit: cost, durability for response, and natural history of disease. In the case of HCV infection, interferon treatment is effective in only about 40%. Since response is usually not permanent, re-treatment and perhaps long-term maintenance therapy is required to maintain control of the disease. Natural history studies have shown that HCV is a slowly progressive disease and that patients at greatest risk of progression are those with moderate to severe periportal inflammation, with or without fibrosis, on their liver biopsy. Therapy is easy to justify in ill patients and those at greatest risk of disease progression. It is also most likely to cost-effective in such patients. On the other hand, therapy, which is likely to be long-term, is difficult to justify in patients with mild histologic disease who would have a low risk of disease progression without treatment. This area is controversial. The observation of higher early response to treatment in patients with minimal disease fuels the argument to initial treatment early, but does not address the high cost of treatment in patients who do not usually require any intervention.

Non-response

Approximately half of all patients will not respond to interferon using a standard regimen. Few alternatives exist for these patients. If the patient has not responded after the first 12 weeks of treatment, escalation of the dose to 10 million units will result in response in about 20% of patients. However, this strategy is associated with the high cost and side effects, and should therefore be reserved for those who have aggressive liver disease or incapacitation symptoms. The emerging role of treatment adjuncts is discussed above.

Relapse

Most patients who respond to treatment will relapse. Although initial reports suggest that as many as only half of responders maintained the initial response to interferon, it is now clear that only 20-30% will maintain normal ALT levels for 6-12 months. Additionally, recent data has suggested that virologic relapse occurs even more commonly and many patients who continue to maintain normal ALT levels may actually be viremic and have active liver disease. These disturbing observations reinforce the need for effective identification of relapse with virologic tools and re-treatment to maintain control of infection and active liver disease. Unfortunately, the best way to treat relapse is not clear. Although almost all patients will again normalize their ALT levels when retreated, it is not clear whether repeated 6 month courses, a titrated long-term maintenance regimen, or some other schedule will best serve the patient. Long-term re-treatment with a fixed dose is clearly not well tolerated and is associated with frequent breakthrough (see below). An international multicenter study (US, Canada, France, Spain, Australia) is currently underway to determine the best way to retreat and maintain remission in interferon-responsive patients.

Breakthrough

In reported trials of interferon, between 0-50% of patients have demonstrated a phenomenon known as breakthrough. Breakthrough occurs in patients who normalized their serum ALT levels in the first weeks of treatment but demonstrate re-evaluation of ALT despite ongoing therapy. It is essentially a relapse during treatment. These episodes are usually associated with reappearance of detectable HCV RNA and appear to be emergence of resistance to the effects of Interferon. The cause of this phenomenon is unclear. Naturalizing anti-Interferon antibodies are responsible for a few cases, particularly with some recombinant Interferon not approved for hepatitis treatment in this country. These cases might also be due to loss of host response to the virus. However, it is likely that most cases result from changes in the virus itself, which render it resistant to the effects of Interferon. This remains to be confirmed.

Definition of Response

The currently accepted definition of response to interferon is normalization of the serum ALT levels at the end of treatment. This definition was arbitrarily defined by investigators in the interferon studies initiated before the identification of the HCV agent. Obviously, documentation of viremia was lacking. The availability of serologic markers of HCV replication (HCV RNA by RT-PCR) confirmed that biochemical response (Normal ALT) was usually associated with a virologic response (negative serum HCV RNA). However, it has recently become apparent that exceptions occur and are associated with early relapse. Additionally, virologic relapse always precedes biochemical relapse, sometimes by months or years. It is clear that the definition of response and relapse needs to be revised to include HCV RNA. Trials are currently underway which will test the appropriateness of various combinations of serologic, biochemical and virologic markers of response, remission, and relapse.

SPECIAL PATIENT GROUPS

Decompensated Cirrhosis

Interferon treatment of decompensated cirrhosis due to hepatitis B is a risky proposition because of the possibility of further decompensation or infection with the flare in ALT, which occurs shortly after beginning treatment. Early experiences with treatment of decompensated cirrhosis due to Hepatitis C indicate that interferon can be administered to most of these patients with good results and no risk of further decompensation (Balart, personal communication).

269

Synthetic function improves in responding patients. Cytopenia and infection may limit therapy in some.

HIV infected patients

HIV co-infected patients have an increased risk of liver failure from chronic Hepatitis C. HCV RNA levels increase over time after HIV seroconversion, particularly once immunodeficiency ensues. HIV and HCV co-infected patients appear to respond no differently to interferon than do patients not infected with HIV, although no study has compared response to HCV RNA levels yet. Thus, Interferon treatment should be considered in HIV co-infected patients before onset of manifestations of immunodeficiency.

Hemophiliacs

Between 60-90% of factor-dependent hemophiliacs have serologic evidence of HCV infection. This occurs because factor concentrates are prepared from plasma pooled from hundreds of individuals who, in many cases, are commercially paid donors. HCV infection is most prevalent in those who have received greater volumes of concentrate, especially of unpasteurized products, and is virtually nonexistent in patients who either have not required factor transfusion of have received exclusively vapor-treated plasma concentrates of recombinant clotting factors. About half of infected patients have abnormal serum ALT levels. Interferon treatment is as effective in this patient population as it is in others and does not appear to be associated with any unique problems. The question of whether or not such patients should have a biopsy before considering treatment is controversial because of the cost and risks of the procedure in these individuals.

Transplant Recipients

HCV infection is common in organ transplant recipients. The true prevalence of infection is considerably underestimated by the tendency for aminotransferase levels to be low to normal and the insensitivity of antibody-based diagnostic tests in immunosuppressed patients. The natural history of HCV infection in transplant recipients is unknown. However, there is a unique syndrome of fibrosing, cholestatic hepatocellular injury similar to that observed in hepatitis B, which occurs in a subset of patients. The role of interferon in treating HCV infection in transplant recipients is not known. Complete response appears to be unusual and there is a small but real risk of acute graft rejection.

Asymptomatic Carriers

Chronic portal or periportal inflammation (CPH or CAH) occurs in 70-100% of anti-HCV and HCV-RNA positive patients with normal ALT levels. In most, the degree of inflammation is mild. Interferon is currently not indicated for these patients for the following reasons: (1) the natural history of the HCV carrier is not known, but is probably comparable to CPH or mild CAH; (2) markers of response to treatment are not available; and (3) most patients are not symptomatic. The possible availability of affordable markers of HCV replication may make treatment based on monitoring viral response feasible in the future.

Extrahepatic Disease

Mixed cryoglobulinemia, membranous glomerulonephritis, and porphyria cutanea tarda may all be associated with HCV infection. In the case of cryoglobulinemia, the cryoglobulins and the associated disease improve or

271

disappear in about half of treated patients. Patients who do not respond to interferon require treatment with immunosuppressive agents including prednisone, cytoxan, and/or pheresis. HCV-associated porphyria responds to phlebotomy. The effects of interferon are not yet described.

TREATMENT OF ACUTE HEPATITIS C

There is a growing consensus that Interferon treatment of acute Hepatitis C reduces the risk of chronicity. Four randomized controlled trials have all demonstrated a reduction in the proportion of patients with either abnormal ALT levels or detectable HCV RNA following a 4-12 week course of Interferon. Although most "responders" maintain their response, some early responders have evidence of infection at a later follow-up. Unfortunately, such patients are rarely identified since acute infection is usually unapparent and it is impractical to serially screen patients with identifiable risk factors.

FUTURE TREATMENT STRATEGIES

Considerable progress has been made in the therapy of chronic hepatitis C in the few years since the identification of this virus. While interferon treatment is quite effective by antiviral standards, there is no doubt that the currently approved regimen is far from optimal. A great deal of work remains in order to better define the clinical guidelines for the use of interferon in patients with chronic Hepatitis C. It is likely that strategies will develop that individualize treatment regimens according to patient characteristics (body size, histology, etc.) and the predominant viral isolate (genotype and level). Better markers of treatment response will allow fine-tuning of the treatment duration and dose. Ongoing trials will hopefully identify the utility of viral markers of response and determine the optimal way to manage the treatment of the infection over the long-term. Finally, new classes of therapeutic agents such as protease inhibitors, antisepses compounds, and therapeutic vaccines will eventually find their way to clinical trials.

REFERENCES
FOR THE TREATMENT OF HEPATITIS C

Standard Therapy

- Hoofnagle, J.H., et al. "Treatment of chronic non-A, non-B hepatitis with recombinant human alpha interferon: A preliminary report." *New Eng. J Med*, 1986; 315:1575-1578.
- Davis, G.L., et al. "Treatment of chronic hepatitis C with recombinant interferon alpha: A multicenter randomized, controlled trial." *New Eng. J Med*, 1989; 321:1501-1506.
- Marcellin P., et al. "Recombinant human alpha-interferon in patients with chronic non A non B hepatitis: a multicenter randomized controlled trial from France." *Hepatology,* 1991; 13:393-397.
- Causse X., et al. "Comparison of 1 or 3 MU of Interferon alfa-2b and placebo in patients with chronic non-A non-B hepatitis." *Gastroenterology,* 1991; 101:497-502.
- Tina F., et al., "Interferon for non-A, non- B chronic Hepatitis: a meta-analysis of randomized clinical trials." *J Hepato,l* 1991; 13:192-199.

Alternative regimens: Higher dose, Longer duration

- Beloqui, O., et al., MP. "N-acetyl cysteine enhances the response to interferon-alpha in chronic hepatitis C: a pilot study." *J Interferon Res*, 1993; 13:279-282.

- Kakumu, S., et al., "A pilot study of ribavirin and interferon beta for the treatment of chronic hepatitis C." *Gastroenterology,* 1993; 105:507- 512.
- Liaw, Y.F., et al., "Effects of prednisone pretreatment in Interferon alfa therapy for patients with chronic non-A, non-B (C) hepatitis." *Liver,* 1993; 13:46-50.

Alternatives to Interferon

- Camps, J., et al., "J. Ribavirin in the treatment of chronic hepatitis C unresponsive to alfa interferon." *J Hepatol,* 1993; 19:408-412.
- Bodenheimer, H.C., et al. "Ribavirin treatment of chronic hepatitis C." *Hepatology* 1994; 20.

SPECIAL PATIENT GROUPS

Decompensated Cirrhosis

- Dimopoulou, M., et al., "Interferon alfa-2a for decompensated liver disease caused by either chronic hepatitis B or C: preliminary results of a pilot study." *Gut* 1993; 34 (suppl. 2): S104-105.

HIV infected patients

- Eyster, M.E., "The natural history of hepatitis C virus infection in multitransfused hemophiliacs: Effects of co-infection with human immuno-deficiency virus." *Acquir Immune Defic Syndr* 1993; 6:602.

- Eyster, M.E., et al., "Increasing HCV RNA levels in hemophiliacs: Relationship to HIV infection and liver disease." *Blood,* 1994.
- Boyer, N., "Recombinant interferon-alpha for chronic hepatitis C in patients positive for antibody to human immunodeficiency virus." *J Infect Dis*, 1992; 165:723-726.

Hemophiliacs

- Makis, M., et al., "A randomized controlled trial of recombinant interferon-alpha in chronic hepatitis C in hemophiliacs." *Blood*, 1991; 78:1672-1677.

Transplant Recipients

- Lim, H.L., et al., "Cholestatic hepatitis leading to hepatic failure in patients with organ- transmitted hepatitis C virus infection." *Gastroenterology*, 1994; 106:248-251.
- Ferrel, L.D., et al., "Hepatitis C viral infection in liver transplant recipients." *Hepatology,* 1992; 16:865-876.
- Wright, H.I., et al., "Preliminary experience with alpha-2b interferon therapy of viral hepatitis in liver allograft recipients." *Transplantation,* 1992; 53:121-124.

Asymptomatic Carriers

- Naito, M., et al., "Serum hepatitis C virus RNA quantity and histological features of hepatitis C virus

carriers with persistently normal ALT levels."
Hepatology, 1994; 19:871-875.

Extrahepatic Disease:

- Lunel, F., et al., "Cryoglobulinemia in chronic liver diseases: role of hepatitis C virus and liver damage." *Gastroenterology*, 1994; 106:1291-1300.

TREATMENT OF ACUTE HEPATITIS C

- Viladomiu, L., et al., "Interferon alpha in acute post transfusion hepatitis C: a randomized controlled trial." *Hepatology*, 1992; 15:767-769.
- Omata, M., et al., "Resolution of acute hepatitis C after therapy with natural beta interferon." *Lancet*, 1991; 338:914-915.
- Lampertico, P., et al., "A multicenter randomized controlled trial of recombinant interferon alpha-2b in patients with acute transfusion- associated hepatitis C." *Hepatology*, 1994; 19:19-22.
- Tassopoulos, N.C., et al. "Recombinant human interferon alfa-2b treatment for acute non-A, non-B hepatitis." *Gut,* 1993; 34:S130-132.

Appendix B

Jackie Judd, ABCNEWS.com, Sept. 17, 1999.

Multiple sclerosis and central nervous disorders can lead to paralysis, slurred speech, and vision problems. While there's no cure, researchers at the Mayo Clinic have developed a treatment that may help people with the most severe cases.

A handful of people, like MS patient Andrew Grant, have already seen the benefits of the new treatment. Though he was completely immobile two years ago, Grant is up and moving again thanks to an experimental approach called plasma exchange.

He and 18 other patients with severely damaged nervous systems had blood removed. A special machine then separated the cells from the plasma, or liquid part of the blood. Plasma from healthy donors was purified until it contained just one protein called albumin. The donor plasma and the original cells were mixed together and put back into the patients.

This exchange was repeated seven times over a two-week period. For this group of severely disabled patients, standard anti-inflammatory treatment hadn't helped. But plasma exchange allowed many of them to regain their speech, as well as movement in their arms and legs.

"We had a robust, major effect in 40 percent of the patients," says Dr. Brian Weinshenker, a Mayo Clinic neurologist and the study's lead researcher.

In those who were helped, the effect was almost immediate.

On day 14, Grant could get out of bed and walk with assistance. Six months later, he could walk on his own.

When he felt his foot move, he says, "I put a big old smile on my face."

Doctors are not entirely sure why this treatment succeeded. An early theory is the patients' plasma contained harmful antibodies that allowed the disease to progress at a rapid pace. The replacement plasma stopped that process.

"I think it's just dramatic," says Weinshenker, "how touching the plasma alone, without doing anything to the cells, can affect an immediate recovery from a neurological disability."

He and his colleagues presented the results of their study, which was funded by the National Institute of Health, at a medical conference today in Basel, Switzerland. They'll publish their findings in the December issue of Annals of Neurology.

The researchers are careful to point out, however, that the new treatment isn't for everyone with MS, and it's not a cure. "Plasma exchange should be considered only for those patients who have severe, acute attacks of MS that are not responsive to high-dose steroid treatments," Weinshenker says.

Appendix C

John McKenzie, ABCNEWS.com, February 28, 2000

It usually begins in medical school when students receive drug company pens, and clocks, and coffee mugs.

When they become doctors, the gifts they receive often increase in value. Drug samples; tickets to ball games; dinners for doctors and their families, even all-expense-paid trips to ski or beach resorts to "consult" with drug company representatives are being given out.

"The companies and sales reps will tell you, " says Dr. Seth Landefeld of the University of California, San Francisco, "you deserve to go out to a particularly nice place, to a nice conference."

It is all part of an intense marketing effort. Each drug company tries to convince doctors of the benefits of its medications, so the doctors, in turn, might prescribe them to you.

By one published estimate, drug companies last year spent an average of $13,000 on every physician in the country, which adds up to more than $8 billion. Drug companies now employ 70,000 sales representatives, which means one sales representative for every nine doctors.

"It is important for pharmaceutical company representatives to be able to help educate doctors about the medicines that the company that discovers and develops them, know best," says Judy Bello, a pharmaceutical industry representative.

The Question is: Do the gifts and entertainment that drug companies offer lead some doctors to practice bad medicine?

"It's the gifts, it's the influence that's the problem," explains Dr. Robert Tenery of the American Medical

Association. "It's creating incentives that may change the way doctors practice medicine and why they prescribe certain medications."

And, potentially, at the patient's expense.

A recent analysis by the Journal of the American Medical Association of 16 different studies showed that doctors courted by drug companies were more likely to engage in "non-rational" prescribing. In other words, they were more likely to order a drug that was more expensive, or less effective, than what the patient actually needed.

The doctors were also more likely -- in some cases, 20 times more likely -- to ask a hospital to add the company's drug to the hospital inventory -- even though most of the requested drugs "presented little or no therapeutic advantage."

Still, most doctors deny that they are influenced by gifts.

"This is a very hot-button issue," says Landefeld. "There are few buttons in medicine you could push that gets doctors stirred up faster."

In part, because many doctors suggest they're too clever to be manipulated by a pharmaceutical company.

"I've worked in places where we've had policies saying we will accept gifts but we won't be influenced by them," says Dr. Allen Shaughnessy of the Medical College of Pennsylvania. "And I try to point out that that's impossible. The two go hand in hand."

The American Medical Association, the country's largest doctor's group, tried to address this problem several years ago. Together with the pharmaceutical industry, the AMA put out guidelines that say gifts to doctors should serve a genuine "educational function" and not be of "substantial" value, usually defined as more than $100.

But these guidelines are voluntary, and the AMA now concedes that many "troubling practices" returned.

APPENDIX D

Influencing Doctors: How Pharmaceutical Companies
Use Enticement to "Educate" Physicians

Brian Ross and David Scott,
ABCNews.com, February 21, 2002

It was doctors' night out last June at the world-renowned Museum of Modern Art in New York City, and the Saturday night party, put on by Pfizer Inc., was lavish.

The event was strictly private, closed to reporters, as the pharmaceutical company entertained a very select list of doctors and their guests. But *Primetime's* undercover cameras saw the kind of big-money splurge that some say drives up the cost of prescription drugs and corrupts the practice of medicine.

Further investigation into the $6 billion spent by drug companies for what they say is a way to educate doctors showed that tactics like lavish gifts and trips are surprisingly common.

"It's embarrassing, it's extravagant and it's unethical," said Dr. Arnold Relman, a Harvard Medical School professor and the former editor of the *New England Journal of Medicine*. "It makes the doctor feel beholden … it suborns the judgment of the doctor."

But doctors seemed thrilled to have been invited for a weekend in New York City with some seminars along the way, with all expenses paid by Pfizer on behalf of one of its drugs, Viagra.

One Small-Town Doctor: $10,000 in Goodies

Few doctors were willing to talk publicly about their relationships with pharmaceutical companies, but one upstate New York doctor was willing to come forward.

"It's very tempting and they just keep anteing it up. And it's getting harder to say no," said Dr. Rudy Mueller. "I feel in some ways it's kind of like bribery."

Disgusted by how the free gifts and trips add to the high price of medicine, and moved by the plight of patients forced to skip needed medication, Mueller agreed to provide *Primetime* with a rare glimpse of the astounding number of drug company freebies he was offered by various drug companies in a four-month period.

He was presented with an estimated $10,000 worth, including an all-expenses-paid trip to a resort in Florida, dinner cruises, hockey game tickets, a ski trip for the family, Omaha steaks, a day at a spa and free computer equipment.

"It changes your prescribing behavior. You just sort of get caught up in it," said Mueller, who said he was offered a cash payment of $2,000 for putting four patients on the latest drug for high cholesterol. The company called this a clinical study; Mueller called it a bounty.

"I've never been offered money before," he said. "I don't remember that 10, 15 years ago."

Though Mueller normally declines the offers, he agreed to attend a dinner, which *Primetime* secretly taped. Not only were the doctors wined and dined, but each was also offered a payment of $150 for just showing up to listen to a pitch for a new asthma treatment for children.

The company called it "an honorarium," but Mueller saw it differently. "Again, it's bribery," he said. "This is very effective marketing."

There's a wide range in value of the free gifts offered to doctors — from lavish trips to free Mother's Day flower bouquets for doctors willing to hear a pitch about a new osteoporosis medicine.

In the latter example, when asked whether a floral shop was the most effective place for a discussion on pharmaceuticals, one of the representatives said, "I'm sorry, we're not allowed to comment on anything."

Detail Men

The goodies are dispensed by an army of drug company representatives known as detail men and women, of whom there are 82,000 nationwide.

It's the job of the detail people to quietly befriend doctors, keeping close track of which doctors take the free gifts and then determining which drugs the doctors later prescribe.

"I think it's sleaze," said Relman. "Anybody who's been in that position knows that yes, those gifts, $60, $100, $40, again and again, do influence your attitude about that company … and will influence the prescriptions that you write."

❄ ❄ ❄

"The American Dream does not end when it comes true for you. It becomes your duty to make it come true for others".

--Dr. David Satcher
Former U.S. Surgeon General

Triumph Over Hepatitis C

A Non-Profit Organization

Tax Deductible Contributions
Product Sales and Ordering
contact Lloyd Wright:

Email: Lloyd@hepatitisCfree.com
Website: www.hepatitiscfree.com
Toll Free 866-IIEPCFREE
(866-437-2373)

As a courtesy to my readers, I am happy to provide
everything in "The Remedy" at wholesale prices.
This is done for your convenience as I had a very
difficult time finding many of the items and was
charged outrageous prices for others.

Thank You for your support!